Endocrinology Research and Clinical Developments

nova
Medicine & Health
New York

Endocrinology Research and Clinical Developments

The Biochemical Guide to Hormones
David Aebisher, PhD, DSc (Editor)
2023. ISBN: 979-8-88697-492-8 (Hardcover)
2023. ISBN: 979-8-88697-534-5 (eBook)

Natural Products for Treatment of Metabolic Syndrome
Ajmer Singh Grewal, PhD (Editors)
Ashwani Kumar Dhingra, PhD (Editors)
2022. ISBN: 979-8-88697-152-1 (Hardcover)
2022. ISBN: 979-8-88697-233-7 (eBook)

A Clinical Guide to Thyroidectomies
Anand Mishra (Editor)
2022. ISBN: 978-1-68507-814-0 (Hardcover)
2022. ISBN: 979-8-88697-033-3 (eBook)

Polycystic Ovary Syndrome: Causes, Diagnosis and Management
Katherine Webb (Editor)
2021. ISBN: 978-1-53619-527-9 (Softcover)
2021. ISBN: 978-1-53619-586-6 (eBook)

Diabetes and Diabetic Complications: Current Status and Future Perspectives
Randhir Singh Dahiya (Editor)
Thakur Gurjeet Singh (Editor)
2021. ISBN: 978-1-53619-177-6 (Hardcover)
2021. ISBN: 978-1-53619-453-1 (eBook)

More information about this series can be found at
https://novapublishers.com/product-category/series/endocrinology-research-and-clinical-developments/

Poongkodi Karunakaran, MCh, PhD
Editor

Understanding and Managing Hyperthyroidism

nova
Medicine & Health
New York

https://doi.org/10.52305/HCEE6098

Library of Congress Cataloging-in-Publication Data

ISBN: 979-8-88697-636-6

Published by Nova Science Publishers, Inc. † New York

Contents

Preface

Understanding and Managing Hyperthyroidism is a comprehensive review of thyroid formative anatomy, physiology, the etiopathogenesis of hyperthyroidism, and current updates in the evaluation and management of thyrotoxic patients. In 1909, Theodor Kocher was awarded the Nobel Prize for his extensive work on thyroid physiology, pathology, and safe surgical techniques. A century later, modern thyroid surgery has undergone a sea of change from conventional open thyroidectomy to remote access robotic scarless thyroidectomy. The chapter on the surgical management of Graves' Disease describes the various thyroid surgical techniques including recent advances. The availability of innovative technology, equipment, training of surgeons, indication for surgery, patient preferences, affordability, and all can influence the operative outcome. This book is intended to serve as a useful resource for endocrine surgeons and endocrinologists as well as guide surgical residents, researchers, clinicians, and general practitioners with a focus of interest on thyroid disease.

Dr. Poongkodi Karunakaran, MCh, PhD

Acknowledgments

I thank all the authors and co-authors for contributing their valuable time and expertise to our book. I thank Dr. Chandrasekaran for his expert guidance and help in coordinating the chapters.

I would also like to thank Donna Dennis and the production team of Nova Science Publishers, Inc, NY, USA.

Chapter 1

Introduction to Hyperthyroidism

Poongkodi Karunakaran, MCh, PhD[1,2,3,*]

[1]Endocrine Surgery Unit, Government Mohan Kumaramangalam Medical College, Salem, India
[2]Department of Endocrine Surgery, Madras Medical College, Chennai, India
[3]The Tamilnadu Dr. MGR Medical University, Chennai, India

Abstract

The thyroid gland is necessary for the optimal maintenance of cellular metabolism and the normal functioning of the cells. Thyrotoxicosis is a constellation of clinical signs and symptoms of hypermetabolism caused by inappropriately high circulating thyroid hormone concentrations, irrespective of source [1]. Hyperthyroidism is a subset of thyrotoxicosis specifically caused by increased production and release of thyroid hormone by the thyroid gland per se [1]. For a better understanding of thyroid disorders and their effective management, a thorough knowledge of the formative anatomy of the thyroid gland and its function is essential. This chapter deals with the historical perspective of the thyroid gland and briefly discusses the anatomy and physiology of the thyroid gland.

Keywords: hyperthyroidism, thyrotoxicosis, overt hyperthyroidism

---

[*] Corresponding Author's Email: poongkodithesurgeon@gmail.com.

In: Understanding and Managing Hyperthyroidism
Editor: Poongkodi Karunakaran
ISBN: 979-8-88697-636-6

1. Introduction

1.1. Historical Perspective

The term "thyroid gland" was introduced by Thomas Wharton in 1656 [2, 3]. The name was derived from a Greek word, "thureos" meaning oblong shield, due to the resemblance of the nearby thyroid cartilage to that of a shield and not by the shape of the thyroid gland itself. Goiter refers to the diffuse enlargement of the thyroid gland. Goiter prevalence and its association with cretinism were known to humankind for centuries. The treatment of goiter with seaweed dates back to 2700 BC, known from Emperor Shen Nung's prescriptions [4]. Ayurveda, a holy script from India, has writings of goiter dating back to 300 BC. In 40 BC, Pliny described goiter prevalence in the Alps and its treatment with burnt seaweed. In 380 AD, Greek Physician Soranus mentioned neck swelling after pregnancy. In 650 AD, Sun Ssu-mo, a Chinese physician, used powdered Mollusks shells and chopped thyroid glands for goiter treatment. In 1500, Leonardo da Vinci first drew the thyroid gland. In 1543, Andreas Vesalius gave the first anatomic description of the thyroid gland. In 1603, Paracelsus first described the association between endemic goiter and congenital idiocy. In 1820, Jean-Francois Coindet first used iodine for the treatment of goiter. Later, in 1873, William Gull first established the causal link between athyreos and cretinism. Caleb Parry was the first to observe the clinical association of palpitation, goiter, and occasionally exophthalmos in spontaneous thyrotoxicosis but believed it to be of cardiac origin. However, his observations were unpublished during his time. In 1835, Robert James Graves, an Irish physician, reported three women with goiter and palpitation and a fourth woman referred by William Stokes with an additional feature of exophthalmos. Coindet reported similar findings in iodine-induced thyrotoxicosis. Later, in 1840, Carl von Basedow formally reported the classic triad of palpitation, goiter, and exophthalmos (Merseburger triad); hence, thyrotoxicosis is still referred Basedow disease in many European countries. The etiology was believed to be of cardiac origin, and in the latter half of the 19th century, it was believed to be of neural etiology rather than the thyroid itself. In 1880, surgeons performed thyroidectomy to treat toxic goiter but with a high mortality rate. However, evidence shows that Abul Kasim of Cordoba first performed a needle biopsy of the thyroid and first described thyroidectomy for goiter in 961 AD. The Swiss surgeon Emil Theodor Kocher employed antisepsis and meticulous surgical techniques to reduce the mortality of thyroidectomy to less than 1%. In 1909, Kocher received the Noble prize for his exemplary work on thyroid gland physiology, pathology, and surgery. Thyroidectomy remained the standard of care for hyperthyroidism until the introduction of 131-I radioactive iodine by Saul Hertz in 1941 and the antithyroid thionamide drug by Edward Astwood in 1943. In 1997, the first endoscopic thyroidectomy was performed, paving the way for minimally invasive surgery and remote-access thyroidectomy. In 2007, Chung performed the first transaxillary robot-assisted thyroidectomy using the Da Vinci Robot system.

2. Embryology of the Thyroid Gland

The thyroid gland has dual embryonic origin from the pharyngeal endoderm and neural crest [5]. The thyroid embryogenesis begins on the 4th week of gestation [5, 6]. The median thyroid anlage evaginates as a diverticulum from the floor of the primitive pharynx, and the foramen caecum represents its vestige remnants at the junction of anterior two-thirds and posterior one-third of the tongue. The diverticulum extends down as a solid column of cells. The distal end bifurcates and becomes bilobed to form the thyroid gland proper. The proximal portion canalizes to form the thyroglossal duct, which later disappears or may persist as a pyramidal lobe for varying lengths. The lateral thyroid anlage from the fourth and fifth pharyngeal pouch unites with the thyroid gland proper on either side posteriorly and contributes to 30% of the thyroid bulk. Zuckerkandl's tubercle, the posterior extension at the junction of the upper and middle third of the lateral lobes of the thyroid, represents the vestigial remnant of the point of fusion of median and lateral anlage. With the pull of the developing heart and extension of the cervical spine, the developing thyroid migrates caudally in front of the foregut. It reaches the final pretracheal position by the seventh month of gestation. The cells show mature thyrocyte differentiation by the tenth week of gestation with the expression of sodium-iodide symporter (NIS), thyroglobulin and thyrotropin receptors. The fetal thyroid begins thyroid hormone synthesis by the 10th or 11th week of gestation and can accumulate radioactive iodine by the eleventh or twelfth week. Neuroectoderm-derived cells migrate through the ultimobranchial bodies and give rise to C cells which produce calcitonin. The superior and inferior parathyroid gland arises from the dorsal portion of the fourth and third pharyngeal pouches, respectively, and comes to lie on the posterior aspect of the lateral lobes of the thyroid.

3. Surgical Anatomy of the Thyroid Gland

The thyroid gland is a bilobed organ with two lateral lobes and a central isthmus, hugging the anterolateral aspects of the larynx and cervical trachea. It occupies the central position in the visceral compartment of the neck just above the thoracic inlet [7]. The thyroid gland extends from the level of the fifth cervical vertebra to the first thoracic vertebra. Each lateral lobe is pyramidal-shaped, measuring roughly 4 cm * 3 cm * 2 cm, and extends from the second to fifth or sixth tracheal rings. The isthmus measures 1 cm * 1 cm and is firmly attached to the second tracheal ring. Pretracheal fascia envelops the gland to form the false capsule or surgical capsule, while the condensation of peripheral thyroid tissues forms the true capsule. The spatium previscerale is the space between the true and false capsule of the gland. This surgical plane allows extracapsular dissection with the identification and preservation of parathyroid glands and recurrent laryngeal nerves. The superior thyroid artery from the external carotid artery and the inferior thyroid artery from the thyrocervical trunk supply the thyroid gland. Three pairs of veins drain the thyroid gland. The superior and middle thyroid vein drains into the internal jugular vein while the inferior thyroid veins drain into the innominate vein. Occasional arteria thyroid ima arising from the arch of the aorta can cause undue hemorrhage during an emergency tracheostomy. The laryngeal nerves do not innervate the thyroid gland but are of surgical importance due to their proximity. Recurrent laryngeal nerves (RLN) arising from the vagus hooks around the right subclavian artery on the right side and ligamentum arteriosum on the left side and ascends in the trachea-esophageal groove. RLN travels behind the posterior surface of the lateral lobe of the thyroid gland and diverges beneath Berry's ligament to enter the larynx under the inferior cornua of the cricoid cartilage. Due to the shorter course, the right RLN ascends with an oblique angle compared to the left RLN, which has a longer intrathoracic course. The external branch of the superior laryngeal nerve travels with the superior thyroid artery. It turns medially near the upper pole of the thyroid to innervate the cricothyroid, which controls the timbre of the voice [8]. The superior parathyroid gland lies dorsolateral to the RLN within 1 cm from the cricothyroid junction above the intersection of RLN and inferior thyroid artery on either side [8, 9]. The inferior parathyroid glands lie ventromedial to the RLN and are inconstant in position due to the longer embryonic descent. A thorough understanding of anatomy is the key to a safe and complete thyroidectomy.

4. Thyroid Physiology

4.1. Hypothalamo-Pituitary Thyroid (HPT) Axis

HPT axis is a classic endocrine negative feedback loop that maintains thyroid hormone levels in the euthyroid range [10, 11]. The paraventricular nucleus synthesizes and secretes thyrotropin-releasing hormone (TRH), which reaches adenohypophysis through the hypothalamo-hypophyseal portal system. TRH acts on pituitary thyrotropes to stimulate the synthesis and release of thyrotropin or thyroid-stimulating hormone (TSH). TSH is a glycoprotein comprising an α-subunit common to all anterior pituitary hormones and a unique β-subunit. TSH acts on thyroid follicular cells to stimulate the cell proliferation and the synthesis and release of 3, 5, 3' triiodothyronine (T3) and 3, 5, 3', 5' tetraiodothyronine (T4). The thyroid hormones, in turn, inhibit the synthesis and release of TRH and TSH at the hypothalamus and pituitary, respectively, thereby completing the negative feedback loop [12]. Thus, TSH has a physiological inverse logarithmic relationship with the thyroid hormones and defines the set-point of the HPT axis. In the physiological milieu, a slight decrease in thyroid hormone levels markedly increases the TSH levels, thereby increasing the synthesis and release of T3 and T4 to achieve euthyroid status and vice versa.

4.2. Thyroid Follicle

The thyroid follicle is the basic functional unit of the thyroid gland. Each follicle is 100μ to 300μ in size and is composed of a single layer of cuboidal epithelial cells surrounding a central lumen filled with colloid. The three essential functions of thyroid follicular cells (TFCs) are 1) Iodine trapping and transport; 2) Thyroglobulin (Tg) synthesis and storage in colloid; 3) Thyroid hormone (TH) synthesis and secretion into the circulation. TFCs synthesize two principal thyroid hormones, thyroxine (T4) and T3. Whereas the neural crest-derived C cells or parafollicular cells in contact with the follicular basement membrane synthesize calcitonin.

4.3. Thyroid Hormone Synthesis and Secretion

Iodine is the principal element essential for TH synthesis. Ingested iodine in the gastrointestinal tract is converted to iodide (I^-) and absorbed into the circulation. The recommended dietary intake of iodine is 150 μg/day in adults, 200 μg/day in pregnant women, and 250 μg/day in lactating mothers to maintain normal thyroid function. The NIS on the basolateral membrane of TFC transports Na^+ and I^- against the electrochemical gradient of iodide and is driven by the Na^+-K^+ ATPase pump. NIS can increase the intrathyroidal iodide concentration to 20-40 times that of plasma. Iodide enters the apical lumen through anion exchanger pendrin (PDS) or other transporters, including anoctamin, cystic fibrosis transmembrane conductance regulator (CFTR), and sodium multivitamin transporter (SMVT) [12]. Tg is a 660kDa glycoprotein exclusively synthesized in the thyroid gland and stored in the colloid (Figure 1). Tg containing 10% carbohydrate and 123 iodotyrosine residues serves as a scaffold for TH synthesis. However, only four to eight tyrosine residues are incorporated into the TH. The thyroperoxidase (TPO) enzyme at the apical membrane of TFCs catalyzes the oxidation of inorganic iodide in the presence of hydrogen peroxidase (H_2O_2). H_2O_2 is generated by dual oxidase (DUOX 1 and 2).

The iodinium ions (I+) or hypoiodous acid or enzyme-linked hypoiodate (E-OI) so formed bind avidly to the 3-position of tyrosine residues of thyroglobulin to form monoiodotyrosine (MIT) and further iodination in the 5-position produces diiodotyrosine (DIT). A coupling reaction is an oxidative condensation of a pair of DIT molecules to form T4, eliminating the alanine side chain from the outer ring molecule. MIT couples with a DIT molecule to produce T3. A small amount of reverse T3 is formed by coupling DIT with the MIT molecule. The same TPO- H_2O_2 enzyme system also catalyzes the coupling reaction. Iodinated Tg (Tg-I) along with TH is engulfed back into the cells by pinocytosis. Lysosomal proteolysis of Tg liberates free T3, free T4, MIT, and DIT into the cytoplasm. The liberated free T3 and free T4 are secreted into circulation mainly by monocarboxylate transporter 8 (MCT8) at a 1:13 ratio (corresponding to that stored in Tg) [13]. MIT and DIT are deiodinated and reutilized for new hormone synthesis. TSH stimulates all the steps involved in TH synthesis, including iodide trapping, oxidation of iodide and organification, coupling reaction, and finally, thyroid hormone release as shown in Figure 1. TSH also stimulates the growth and proliferation of the TFCs. In the quiescent phase, TFCs are cuboidal or flat distended with colloid. Whereas TSH-stimulated TFCs are tall and columnar with virtually absent colloid. Transcription factors including Tiff1, Foxe 1, Pax8, and Hhex are involved in the transcription of genes encoding NIS, TPO, Tg, and TSH receptors. Thioureas and thioimidazoles bind to TPO and inhibit iodine oxidation, iodination of tyrosyl residues, and coupling reactions, thereby inhibiting TH synthesis. Whereas, Iodides inhibit TH release and are hence known as thyroid constipators.

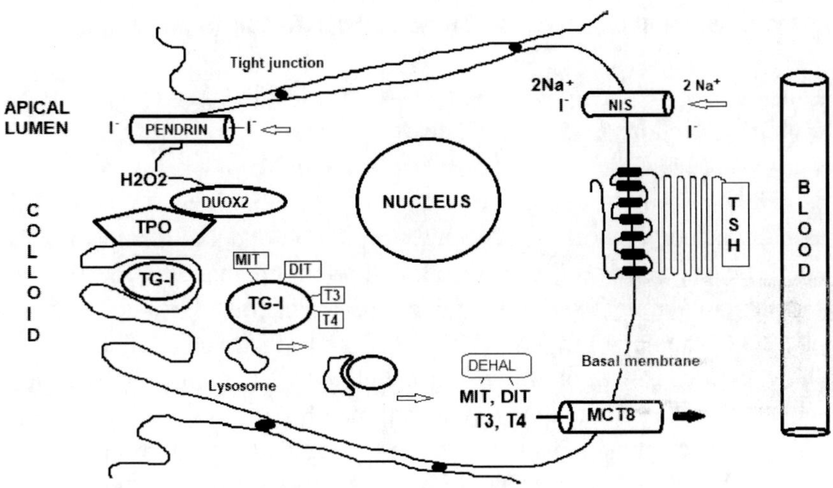

Figure 1. Thyroid hormone synthesis in thyroid follicular cells. The sodium-iodide symporter along the basolateral membrane traps iodide, which diffuses through the pendrin channel into the apical lumen. The oxidation of iodide at the apical-colloidal interface by the thyroperoxidase enzyme (TPO), requires the substrate hydrogen peroxide generated by dual oxidase (DUOX). TPO also catalyzes the iodination of tyrosyl residues of thyroglobulin. The coupling of two DIT and one MIT with DIT produces T4 and T3 which remains attached to thyroglobulin in the colloid. Colloidal uptake of iodinated thyroglobulin (TG-I) and lysosomal proteolysis liberates T3, T4, MIT, and DIT. T3 and T4 enter the bloodstream through monocarboxylate transporter 8 (MCT8). TSH stimulates all the steps involved in thyroid hormone synthesis.

4.4. Thyroid Hormone Transport and Metabolism

The normal human thyroid secretes about 80 μg of T4, 4 μg of T3, and 2 μg of rT3 daily. In adults, the total plasma T4 level is about 8 μg/dL with a half-life of 7 days, while plasma T3 levels are 0.15 μg/dL with a plasma half-life of 8-12 hours [14]. More than 99% of the circulating TH are protein-bound, and only 0.03 to 0.08% of T4 and 0.2% to 0.5% of T3 are in the free form.

The plasma proteins that bind TH are thyroid-binding globulin, transthyretin, and albumin, in the order of decreasing affinity. Only the free forms are available for hormone action, metabolism, and excretion. T3 and T4 are inactivated by deiodination in the liver and kidney. TH and its deiodinated derivatives undergo glucuronide or sulfate conjugation and are excreted in the bile. A significant fraction is deconjugated in the intestine, reabsorbed (in enterohepatic circulation), and ultimately excreted in the urine. In hyperthyroidism, the half-lives are shortened due to a faster metabolism.

4.5. Peripheral Conversion of T4 to T3

T4 is 99.97% protein-bound and acts as a prohormone. Whereas the biologically active T3 hormone is 99.7% protein-bound and 0.3% is the free fraction. The circulating T4 is three to four-fold higher than the free T3 level. Most of the circulating T3 is generated by the peripheral conversion of T4 by type 1 iodothyronine deiodinase (DIO), mainly in the liver and kidney. The lipophilic TH diffuses through the cell membrane of the target cells to reach the nucleus and is facilitated by special cell membrane transporters, including monocarboxylate transporter-8 (MCT-8), MCT-10, and organic acid transporter protein 1c1 (OATP1c1). The availability and binding of intracellular active T3 to nuclear thyroid hormone receptor (TR) is determined by the relative activity of type 2 and type 3 deiodinase enzymes (DIO2 and DIO3). DIO2 converts T4 to active T3 by the removal of a 5'-iodine atom. DIO3 converts T4 to inactive metabolites, rT3 (3,3',5'-triiodothyronine) and T2 (diiodothyronine). Pre-receptor T3 availability controls the magnitude and timing of the tissue-specific target cell responses. Most target cells take up T3 depending on their metabolic needs, except for the brain, which takes up T4 and converts it to T3 within its own cells. Propylthiouracil (not carbimazole), high dose propranolol, amiodarone, and glucocorticoids inhibit the peripheral conversion of T4 to T3.

4.6. Mechanism of Action of Thyroid Hormones

The thyroid hormone receptor (TR) belongs to the steroid receptor superfamily. Four isoforms of TR, including TRα1, TR α2, TRβ1, and TRβ2, are formed by the differential splicing of THRA and THRB genes located on chromosomes 17 and 3, respectively. Unliganded TRs mediate transcriptional repression of the target genes. The binding of T3 to these nuclear receptors results in derepression and activation of the gene transcription of T3-responsive elements. TRα1 and TRβ1 are expressed in most cells, but the relative concentration is cell-specific. TRβ2 mediates negative feedback regulation in the hypothalamus and pituitary. TR α2 does not bind ligands, and little is known about its function.

5. Overt and Subclinical Hyperthyroidism

Overt hyperthyroidism is characterized by the clinical manifestation of thyrotoxicosis with elevated free T3 and/or free T4 levels despite suppressed TSH. In subclinical hyperthyroidism, patients are asymptomatic with normal free T3 and free T4 levels but suppressed TSH levels. Graves' disease is the most common cause of hyperthyroidism, followed by toxic multinodular goiter and toxic adenoma. The etiopathogenesis, clinical presentation, diagnosis, and management of hyperthyroidism will be described in subsequent chapters.

Conclusion

The hypothalamo-pituitary thyroid axis is a classical negative feedback loop that maintains euthyroid status. TSH has an inverse logarithmic relationship with thyroid hormones. Thyrotoxicosis is a clinical syndrome of hypermetabolism caused by excess circulating thyroid hormones. Hyperthyroidism is a subset of thyrotoxicosis specifically caused by increased synthesis and release of thyroid hormones by the thyroid gland.

References

[1] de Leo S, Lee SY, Braverman LE. Hyperthyroidism. *The Lancet* 2016;388:906–18. https://doi.org/10.1016/S0140-6736(16)00278-6.

[2] Cornelius Medvei V. *The history of clinical endocrinology: A comprehensive account of endocrinology from earliest times to the present day*. 1993.

[3] Kopp P. The heritage of thyroid: A brief history. In: Braverman LE, Cooper DS, Kopp P, editors. *Werner & Ingbar's The Thyroid: A Fundamental and Clinical Text,*

vol. 1. 11th ed., Philadelphia: Lippincott Williams & Wilkins (LWW); 2021, p. 1–8.

[4] Sawin Clark T. *Thyroid History Timeline: The Clark T. Sawin History Resource Center*. American Thyroid Association n.d. https://www.thyroid.org/about-american-thyroid-association/clark-t-sawin-history-resource-center/thyroid-history-timeline/(accessed July 7, 2022).

[5] Henry Jean Francois. Surgical anatomy and embryology of the thyroid and parathyroid glands and recurrent and external laryngeal nerves. In: Clark OH, Duh Q-Y, Kebebew E, Gosnell JE, Shen WT, editors. *Textbook of Endocrine Surgery*. Third, Philadelphia: The Health Sciences Publishers; 2016, p. 11–22.

[6] Agarwal A, Mishra AK, Lombardi CP, Raffaelli M. Applied Embryology of the Thyroid and Parathyroid Glands. In: Randolph GW, editor. *Surgery of the Thyroid and Parathyroid Glands*. 2nd ed., USA: Elsevier Saunders; 2013, p. 15–24.

[7] Decker GAG, du Plessis DJ. The thyroid, thymus and the parathyroid gland. In: Decker DJ, editor. *Lee McGregor's Synopsis of Surgical Anatomy*. 12th ed., Bristol: John Wright & Sons Ltd.; 1986, p. 198–205.

[8] Mohebati A, Shaha AR. Anatomy of thyroid and parathyroid glands and neurovascular relations. *Clinical Anatomy* 2012;25. https://doi.org/10.1002/ca.21220.

[9] Bliss RD, Gauger PG, Delbridge LW. Surgeon's Approach to the Thyroid Gland: Surgical Anatomy and the Importance of Technique. *World Journal of Surgery* 2000;24. https://doi.org/10.1007/s002680010173.

[10] Bassett JHD, Williams GR. Role of Thyroid Hormones in Skeletal Development and Bone Maintenance. *Endocrine Reviews* 2016;37:135–87. https://doi.org/10.1210/er.2015-1106.

[11] Braverman LE, Cooper DS, Kopp P, editors. *Werner & Ingbar's The Thyroid: A Fundamental and Clinical Text*. vol. 1. 11th ed. Philadelphia: Lippincott Williams & Wilkins (LWW); 2021.

[12] Kopp PA. Thyroid Hormone Synthesis. In: Braverman LE, Cooper DS, Kopp PA, editors. *Werner & Ingbar's The Thyroid: A Fundamental and Clinical Text,* vol. 1. 11th ed., Cooper, David S: Lippincott Williams & Wilkins (LWW); 2021, p. 59–85.

[13] Clifton-Bligh R, Delbridge LW. Thyroid Physiology. In: Clark HO, Duh Q-Y, Kebebew E, Gosnell JEsWT, editors. *Textbook of Endocrine Surgery*. 3rd ed., Philadelphia: Jaypee Brothhers Medical Publishers; 2016, p. 3–10.

[14] Barret KE, Barman SM, Boitano S, Brooks HL. Ganong, *Wf - Review of Medical Physiology*. 2016.

Chapter 2

The Epidemiology and Etiopathogenesis of Graves' Disease

Melina Saban[1,*]
Marina Inés Curria[1,†]
Horacio Romeo[2,‡]
and María Laura Barreiro Arcos[2,§]

[1]Division of Endocrinology, Metabolism, Nutrition and Diabetes, British Hospital of Buenos Aires, Buenos Aires, Argentina
[2]School of Engineering and Agrarian Sciences, Pontifical Catholic University of Argentina (UCA), Institute of Biomedical Research (BIOMED-UCA-CONICET), Buenos Aires, Argentina

Abstract

Graves' disease (GD) is the most common cause of hyperthyroidism. GD is an endocrine autoimmune disorder caused by the presence in serum of TSH receptor-stimulating autoantibodies (TRAb) that induce the overproduction of 3, 5, 3'-triiodo-L-thyronine (T3) and L-thyroxine (T4) and enlargement of the thyroid gland. GD is also often accompanied by autoantibodies against other thyroid antigens such as thyroglobulin and thyroid peroxidase. The prevalence of GD is around 1-1.5% worldwide, with an incidence of 20 to 50 new cases per 100,000 inhabitants per year with a considerably higher frequency in women than in men. In addition

[*] Corresponding Author's Email: sabanmelina@gmail.com.
[†] Corresponding Author's Email: marinacurria@gmail.com.
[‡] Corresponding Author's Email: horacio_romeo@uca.edu.ar.
[§] Corresponding Author's Email: mlbarreiro@yahoo.com.ar.

In: Understanding and Managing Hyperthyroidism
Editor: Poongkodi Karunakaran
ISBN: 979-8-88697-636-6

to hyperthyroidism, extrathyroidal manifestations including orbitopathy, thyroid dermopathy, and acropachy are frequently associated with GD.

Genetic factors (such as HLA-DR3, CD40, CTLA-4, PTPN22, *FOXP3,* and CD25) and environmental and endogenous factors (such as age, emotional stress, smoking, female sex, pregnancy, bacterial and viral infections, and some drugs) contribute to the development of GD.

Although the pathogenesis of GD has been better understood, directed treatments against the molecular mechanisms are lacking. Therapies for GD are presently based upon antithyroid drugs, but due to the high rate of recurrence in hyperthyroidism, ablation of the thyroid by either radioiodine treatment or surgical thyroidectomy is the only treatment available.

In the present chapter, we provide updated knowledge on the epidemiology and etiopathogenesis of GD.

Keywords: Graves' disease, autoimmunity, thyroid gland, thyroid hormones, orbitopathy, epidemiology, etiopathogenesis

1. Introduction

Graves' disease (GD), also called Graves-Basedow disease, is an autoimmune endocrine pathology characterized by goiter, hyperthyroidism, and orbitopathy. It was first described in 1835 by the Irish physician Robert James Graves and later, in 1840, by the German physician Karl Adolph von Basedow [1].

It is widely distributed worldwide, with a higher prevalence in women than men. Although between ages 30 and 60 years are more frequent, the disease may develop at any time in life [2].

During this autoimmune disease, patients manifest symptoms and signs typical of hyperthyroidism [3]. For several decades the mechanisms of action remained unknown. Current knowledge attributes the disease to a deregulation of the immune system that induces the aberrant production of autoantibodies directed against the thyroid-stimulating hormone receptor (TSH-R) expressed on the follicular epithelial cells of the thyroid gland [3]. Moreover, the exact pathogenic mechanisms are not fully elucidated as Graves' disease is multifactorial, involving genetic, endogenous, and environmental factors [1].

In this chapter, the epidemiology of GD will be analyzed, and the risk factors and molecular mechanisms involved in the development and progression of the disease will be discussed.

2. Epidemiology of Graves' Disease

2.1. Clinical Manifestations

GD is an autoimmune endocrine disorder caused by antibodies against the TSH-R, mimicking the action of thyroid-stimulating hormone (TSH) and causing hyperfunction of the gland that leads to hyperthyroidism [3].

Most of the signs and symptoms of GD are caused by the direct and indirect effects of hyperthyroidism on tissues, the main exceptions being orbitopathy, goiter, pretibial myxedema (localized dermopathy), and acropachy of the fingers or toes, which are caused by autoimmune processes [3].

The most common symptoms caused by hyperthyroidism are fatigue, insomnia, hand tremors, hyperactivity, hair loss, excessive sweating, warm and moist skin, heat intolerance, weight loss despite increased appetite, oligomenorrhea, diarrhea, frequent defecation, palpitations, and muscle weakness. The most frequent signs observed on physical examination of patients are diffuse and symmetrical enlargement of the thyroid gland (goiter), orbitopathy, and cardiac abnormalities such as arrhythmias, sinus tachycardia, atrial fibrillation, premature ventricular contractions, and hypertension [2, 3].

Cardiovascular alterations are the major and serious complications of hyperthyroidism in GD. In fact, about 80% of patients display tachycardia, and 50% have high blood pressure. Untreated hyperthyroidism can lead to cardiovascular disease and even death. Therefore, the diagnosis and treatment of the pathology must be carried out promptly [4].

Orbitopathy is the most common extrathyroidal manifestation of GD. About 25-50% of patients with Graves' disease develop it, a condition characterized by periorbital edema, proptosis (exophthalmos) with eyelid retraction, extraocular muscle dysfunction (lid lag), and excessive lacrimation, impairing the quality of life of patients [5, 6]. In 5-10% of patients with Graves' orbitopathy, the inflammation of the ocular orbit is so intense that diplopia occurs. The most severe manifestation of this process is the compression of the optic nerve, which can lead to unavoidable and permanent vision loss. Hyperthyroidism followed by orbitopathy typically occurs within a year but also can be separated by decades. GD also causes behavioral and personality changes, comprising psychosis, nervousness, anxiety, and depression [7].

2.2. Epidemiological Data

GD is the most common cause of hyperthyroidism in developed countries, with a prevalence of overt hyperthyroidism of 0.2-1.3% worldwide and an incidence of 20 to 50 new cases per 100,000 persons per year. About 60-80% of patients with hyperthyroidism are diagnosed with Graves' disease [8].

The incidence of GD depends on the iodine intake of the population. The prevalence of GD is higher in geographic areas with iodine deficiency [8]. Patients with endemic goiter due to iodine deficiency or patients with GD who are clinically euthyroid develop hyperthyroidism when more iodine becomes available, an effect known as Jod-Basedow's effect. Several authors have described incidence values in different countries, even among geographic regions of the same country, with significant differences. These changes in incidence may reflect improved detection as the result of an improvement in methods of diagnosis rather than actual changes in the incidence rates or may reflect the impact of differences in iodine intake [9, 10].

Approximately 3% of women and 0.5% of men develop GD during their lifetime. The peak incidence of GD occurs among patients aged 30 to 60, but people can be affected at any age. The incidence in women is 8 to 10-fold higher than in men and probably results from the influence of genetic and hormonal factors. Even in children, where the pathology is less frequent, a female preponderance is about tenfold higher to develop GD compared to the male gender [1, 11].

The annual incidence of Graves' orbitopathy is 16 cases per 100,000 women and 3 cases per 100,000 men [6].

3. Etiopathogenesis of Graves' Disease

3.1. Hypothalamic-Pituitary-Thyroid Axis and Synthesis of Thyroid Hormones

The thyroid gland is the endocrine organ where the thyroid hormones thyroxine (T4) and 3, 5, 3′ triiodothyronine (T3) are synthesized and stored. It is located in the anterior region of the neck and consists of two symmetrical lobes attached to the sides of the trachea and larynx. Histologically, the gland presents follicles of variable size constituted by a monolayer of cylindrical epithelial cells around a central lumen containing colloid. Thyroid follicles are the functional structures that synthesize, store and secrete T3 and T4 [12]. The steps by which the follicles synthesize and secrete thyroid hormones are described below and in Figure 1.

The synthesis of T3 and T4 begins with the uptake of iodide by thyroid follicular cells from the bloodstream through the NIS transporter located in the basal membrane. The iodide then enters the colloid via the pendrin carrier protein located in the apical membrane and is oxidized by thyroid peroxidase (TPO) using endogenously generated hydrogen peroxide. Thyroglobulin (TG), a high molecular weight dimeric glycoprotein, is synthesized, glycosylated, and packaged into secretory granules that are released into the follicle lumen by exocytosis. In the follicular lumen, TPO catalyzes two essential steps in the synthesis of thyroid hormones, the progressive iodination of tyrosine residues in TG to form monoiodinated (MIT) or di-iodinated (DIT) iodotyrosines, a process known as organification of the TG and, the coupling of two iodotyrosines to form thyroglobulin-bound iodothyronines. The iodothyronines are stored in the follicular lumen as colloids and are then endocytosed by thyroid follicular cells, a process stimulated by TSH. Within the follicular cells, endocytic vesicles containing iodinated TG bind to lysosomes where the hormones T4 and T3 are released from the TG by endopeptidases. The thyroid hormones then reach the bloodstream through specific transporters in the thyroid cells [2, 12]. The thyroid gland synthesizes and secretes much more T4 than T3. About 80% of the T3 in the bloodstream results from monodeiodination of T4 in peripheral tissues by deiodinases [12].

Thyroid hormones regulate the metabolism of proteins, carbohydrates, and lipids and participate in several physiological processes that regulate the functioning of the nervous system, bone and muscle development, reproduction, and tissue differentiation. Due to the pleiotropic actions of thyroid hormones in most tissues, precise control of the synthesis and secretion of T3 and T4 by the thyroid gland is essential. Thus, the physiological levels of thyroid hormones in the bloodstream and tissues result from a strict regulation system mediated by the hypothalamic-pituitary-thyroid axis [12].

In response to decreased T3 and T4 levels in the bloodstream and tissues, the hypothalamus synthesizes and secretes a tripeptide called thyrotropin-releasing hormone (TRH) that binds to specific receptors on the thyrotropin cells of the anterior pituitary or adenohypophysis, stimulating the production and release of TSH. TSH, a low molecular weight glycoprotein, then binds to receptors on thyroid follicular cells and induces different processes such as

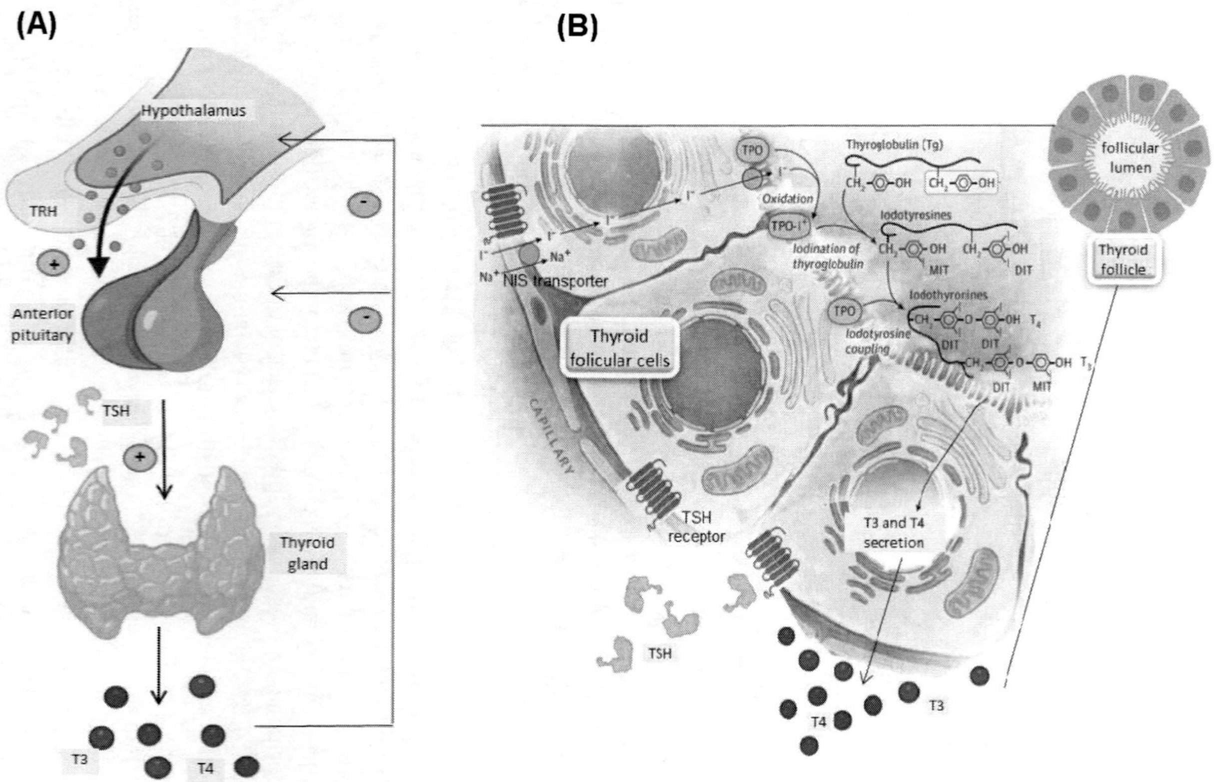

Figure 1. (A) Hypothalamic-pituitary-thyroid axis. The hypothalamic-pituitary-thyroid axis regulates the levels of thyroid hormones in the bloodstream and tissues. When T3 and T4 levels are decreased, the hypothalamus synthesizes and secretes the TRH that binds to

specific receptors on the thyrotropin cells of the anterior pituitary, stimulating the production and release of TSH. TSH, then binds to receptors on thyroid follicular cells, stimulating the synthesis and secretion of thyroid hormones. In response to increased levels of T3 and T4 (above physiological values), thyroid hormones exert negative feedback control on the hypothalamus and anterior pituitary, inhibiting the release of both TRH and TSH, which restores the physiological values of thyroid hormones in the bloodstream and tissues. (B) Thyroid hormone biosynthesis. The synthesis of T3 and T4 begins with the uptake of iodide by thyroid follicular cells from the bloodstream through the NIS transporter. The iodide then enters the colloid and is oxidized by TPO using endogenously generated hydrogen peroxide. TPO catalyzes two essential steps in the synthesis of thyroid hormones, the progressive iodination of tyrosine residues in TG to form monoiodinated (MIT) or di-iodinated (DIT) iodotyrosines and, the coupling of two iodotyrosines to form thyroglobulin-bound iodothyronines. The iodothyronines are stored in the follicular lumen as colloids and are then endocytosed by thyroid follicular cells, a process stimulated by TSH. Within the follicular cells, T4 and T3 are released from TG and enter the bloodstream.

iodide uptake by the NIS transporter and iodination and proteolysis of TG stimulating the synthesis and secretion of thyroid hormones. In response to increased levels of T3 and T4 (above physiological values), thyroid hormones exert negative feedback control on the hypothalamus and anterior pituitary, inhibiting the release of both TRH and TSH, which restores the physiological concentrations of thyroid hormones in the bloodstream and tissues [12]. The hypothalamic-pituitary-thyroid axis and its regulation by thyroid hormones are depicted in Figure 1.

Thyroid hormone levels above or below physiological concentrations as a result of dysregulation of the hypothalamic-pituitary-thyroid axis can lead to states of overt hyperthyroidism or hypothyroidism, respectively. Subclinical forms of these disorders have also been defined, characterized by a reduction or increase in circulating TSH depending on whether it is subclinical hyperthyroidism or hypothyroidism. As their names indicate, the symptoms of the disease are mild or absent but can progress to overt hyperthyroidism or hypothyroidism if treatment is not given [13].

Hyperthyroidism in GD results from the action of autoreactive immunoglobulins that stimulate the TSH-R on thyroid follicular cells. The levels of these autoantibodies directed against the TSH-R (TRAb) correlate with the severity of the disease and probably cause Graves' orbitopathy by binding to TSH-R that are expressed in retroorbital tissues [14].

3.2. Pathogenic Mechanisms in the Development of Graves' Disease

GD begins as a result of the breakdown of immunological tolerance towards self-thyroid antigens, thus initiating an autoimmune process. The causes are multifactorial, involving polygenic, environmental, or endogenous components [1].

Patients with GD have significant concentrations of TRAb and progressive infiltration of the thyroid gland by T and B lymphocytes [3]. Stimulating TRAb mimics the actions of TSH; they activate the TSH-R continuously (even when TSH levels are low or undetectable), inducing thyroid follicular cell hypertrophy and hypersecretion of T3 and T4. Although, to a lesser extent, TRAb blockers capable of inducing hypothyroidism have been found. Thyroid activity is the result of the balance between the action of stimulating and blocking antibodies [3, 15]. In addition, antibodies directed against other thyroid antigens such as thyroglobulin (anti-TG) and thyroid peroxidase (TPOAb) are frequently detected in patients with GD. However, unlike TRAb, these antibodies are not specific for GD, and their determination in plasma is not used as a method of diagnosing the disease [3, 16]. Stimulating antibodies directed against insulin-like growth factor 1 (IGF-1) receptor, which are involved in the development of Graves' orbitopathy, have also been detected in patients with GD [3, 17].

The molecular mechanisms by which autoantibodies directed against thyroid antigens are produced begin with the breakdown of immunological tolerance and the spread of autoreactive T cells from central thymic and peripheral editing [3]. Autoreactive T lymphocytes ($CD4^+$ helper T cells) interact with TSH-R peptides presented on MHC class II molecules by antigen-presenting cells and then differentiate into effector T cells [3]. Intrathyroid T cells are particularly reactive to thyroid antigens and predominantly have the Th2 phenotype. However, the question of whether Graves' disease is biased to the Th1 (cell mediated immunity) or Th2 (humoral immunity) functional subset remains controversial [18]. Autoreactive effector T cells can then activate B cell proliferation and differentiation into plasma cells that produce antibodies directed against thyroid antigens. The oligoclonal production of antibodies against the TSH-R correlates with the degree of lymphocytic infiltrate in the thyroid tissue and with the severity of the pathology [3, 19].

The mechanisms of activation of autoreactive T and B cell clones are complex. They involve the aberrant interaction between lymphocyte cells, signaling coactivator molecules, and the action of cytokines and chemokines produced by antigen-presenting cells and lymphocyte cells. These mechanisms are summarized in Figure 2A.

The involvement of follicular epithelial cells in the pathogenesis of GD has been described, although their role in autoimmunity has not been fully elucidated. These cells express thyroid antigens such as TSH-R, TG, and TPO, and they can secrete several chemokines resulting in the recruitment of immune cells [20]. Furthermore, in patients with GD, thyroid epithelial cells express MHC class II molecules, probably due to the action of interferon-γ produced by infiltrating lymphocytes in thyroid tissue [21]. Thus, although thyroid epithelial cells are not professional antigen-presenting cells, they have the potential to present thyroid antigens to autoreactive T cells. In addition, these cells express the coactivator molecule CD40, essential for the activation of T cells [22]. Thus, thyroid epithelial cells could play a secondary role in the pathogenesis of GD after autoreactive lymphocytes have infiltrated thyroid tissue.

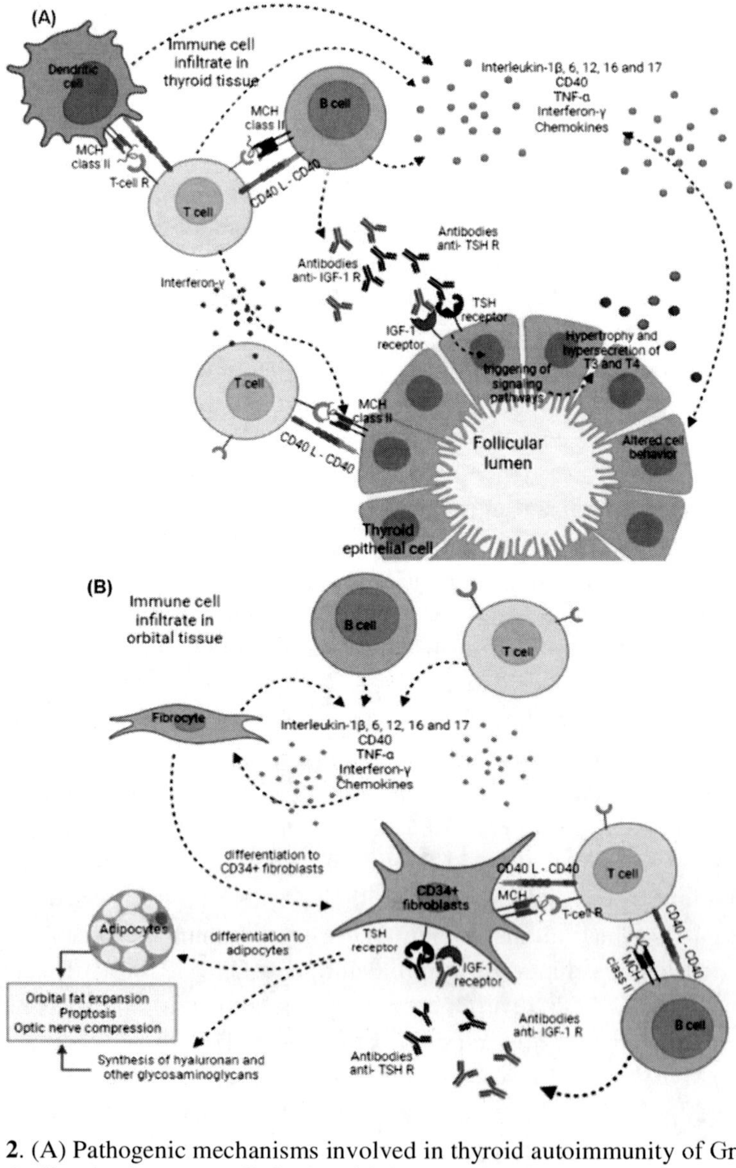

Figure 2. (A) Pathogenic mechanisms involved in thyroid autoimmunity of Graves' disease. Infiltrating immune cells in thyroid tissue such as B and T cells and antigen-presenting cells produce interleukin 1β, 6, 12, 16 and 17, interferon γ, tumor necrosis factor α (TNF-α), CD40 ligand (CD40L) and other cytokines. These inflammatory mediators regulate activation signals of T and B cells and alter the behavior of thyroid epithelial cells. Effector T cells against self-thyroid antigens activate B cell proliferation and their differentiation into antibody-producing plasma cells. Antibodies against the TSH-R secreted by these B cells, mimic the actions of TSH

and induce thyroid follicular cell hypertrophy and hypersecretion of T3 and T4. Autoantibodies against IGF-1 receptor, also participate in signaling pathways that lead to follicular cell hypertrophy, although the underlying mechanisms are unclear. Thyroid epithelial cells express the thyroid antigens TSH-R, TG and TPO and, secrete several chemokines resulting in the recruitment of immune cells. These cells also express MHC class II molecules, probably as a result of the action of interferon-γ produced by infiltrating lymphocytes in thyroid tissue, and then they have the potential to present thyroid antigens to autoreactive T cells. (B) Pathogenic mechanisms involved in Graves' orbitopathy. The orbit is infiltrated by B and T cells and fibrocytes. The bone marrow-derived fibrocytes differentiate into CD34+ fibroblasts, which can further differentiate into adipocytes. CD34+ fibroblast coinhabit the orbit with residential $CD34^-$ fibroblasts. These cell types produce interleukin 1β, 6, 12, 16 and 17, TNF-α, interferon γ, RANTES, and CD40L that induce the activation of $CD34^+$ fibroblasts. The $CD34^+$ fibroblast express low levels of thyroid antigens that can be efficiently presented to T cells, establishing an aberrant immune response. Autoreactive B cells produce antibodies against TSH and IGF-1 receptors that activate their receptors on fibroblasts, inducing the secretion of cytokines, synthesis of hyaluronan and other glycosaminoglycans, and adipogenesis. These events cause expansion of the orbital tissue and extraocular muscle fibers, proptosis, and compression of the optic nerve.

Graves' orbitopathy shares similar immune mechanisms with thyroid autoimmunity. The orbit is infiltrated by autoreactive T and B cells and circulating bone marrow-derived fibrocytes. These cell types produce molecular mediators such as interleukins 1, 6, 8, and 16, tumor necrosis factor (TNF-α), RANTES (regulated upon activation, normal T-cell expressed and secreted), and CD40 involved in the differentiation and activation of fibrocytes to proinflammatory $CD34^+$ fibroblasts [23, 24].

$CD34^+$ fibroblasts express thyroid antigens such as TSH-R, TG, and TPO, which in previous decades were thought to be restricted to the thyroid gland. These antigens can be efficiently presented by fibroblasts to T cells through molecular interactions involving the MHC, CD40, and CD40L molecules and the T-cell receptor TCR. In addition, overexpression of the IGF-1 receptor has been found in the orbital fibroblasts of patients with GD [25]. Both the IGF-1 receptor and TSH-R, expressed in the membrane of fibroblasts, have a functional and physical relationship since it has been proven that the inhibition of signaling by IGF-1 attenuates signaling downstream of TSH-R [25, 26].

Infiltrating B lymphocytes in orbital tissue produce antibodies against TSH and IGF-1 receptors, demonstrating the relevance of these signaling pathways in the autoimmune etiology of GD. Activation of these receptors induces the production of cytokines, hyaluronan, and other glycosaminoglycans and adipogenesis due to the proliferation of adipocytes derived from $CD34^+$ fibroblasts [27, 28]. As a result, there is an expansion of the orbital tissue and extraocular muscle fibers, proptosis, and compression of the optic nerve, which characterize the orbitopathy of GD. With disease progression, the extraocular muscles may also become fibrotic, resulting in restricted mobility [5-7]. The autoimmune mechanisms involved in GD orbitopathy are summarized in Figure 2B.

Conventional treatments for GD reduce the symptoms of the disease by restoring thyroid hormone levels to euthyroidism, but their action is not directed towards immunological targets involved in the aberrant immune response against self-antigens.

The therapeutic treatment of GD involves the use of the antithyroid drugs methimazole (MMI) or propylthiouracil (PTU) with inhibitory action on the production of T3 and T4 in the thyroid gland due to their interference in iodine uptake. PTU also inhibits peripheral conversion of T4 to T3 in tissues but cannot be used in patients with liver failure or pregnancy. MMI is the first-line treatment for the management of hyperthyroidism in GD due to its greater long-term effectiveness and a lower rate of adverse effects [29]. Complementary to treatment with antithyroid drugs, a β-blocker is used to control adrenergic activity, such as atenolol or propranolol. Treatment with antithyroid drugs has a high rate of recurrence of hyperthyroidism, thus thyroid ablation by radioactive iodine or thyroidectomy is necessary [29].

In recent years, drugs with direct action on molecular targets involved in the regulation of the immune response have been developed in order to reduce the activity of autoreactive T and B lymphocytes against thyroid antigens. New therapeutic strategies based on the control of the immune response have shown promising results.

4. Risk Factors in the Development of Graves' Disease

GD is caused by the breakdown of immunological tolerance towards self-antigens of the thyroid gland. The autoimmune process induces the production of TRAb by clones of B cells that infiltrate the thyroid gland [3].

Stimulating TRAb induces hyperthyroidism by activating TSH-R on thyroid cells. The breakdown of immunological tolerance also induces the production of TPOAb and/or TGAb in 50 to 70% of cases of GD [16].

GD risk factors have not been fully defined. The development of this autoimmune disease is multifactorial, involving a complex interaction between endogenous, environmental, and genetic factors.

4.1. Genetic Factors

The genetic predisposition accounts for about 79% of the risk of GD, while endogenous and environmental factors account for 21% [11]. Abundant epidemiological data, including family and twin studies, point to a strong genetic influence on the development of autoimmune thyroid diseases. The genetic susceptibility might explain the ethnic differences in the prevalence of GD.

About 70% of the genes known to correlate with GD risk are involved in T-cell function, indicating the involvement of T-lymphocytes in the pathogenesis of autoimmune thyroid diseases. Next-generation sequencing (NGS) studies and bioinformatic analyzes have identified many predisposing genes involved in GD [11].

The predisposition to GD is polygenic, requiring the co-expression of several gene polymorphisms for an increased risk of GD. Among the genes correlated to GD are those that participate in immunoregulatory functions such as human leukocyte antigens (HLA), cytotoxic T lymphocyte-associated antigen 4 (CTLA-4), CD40, protein tyrosine phosphatase-22 (PTPN 22), CD25 and *FOXP3*, and those related to thyroid physiology as TSH-R and TG [1, 11].

4.1.1. Immunomodulatory Genes

GD is considered an HLA class II-associated pathology. HLA class II expression is polygenic and is encoded by several genes called HLA-DP (A/B), HLA-DQ (A/B), HLA-DRα, and HLA-DRβ (DRB1 and DRB3) [30]. These genes are polymorphic expressing multiple variants or alleles. Individuals have two sets of HLA alleles or haplotypes, as a result of paternal and maternal chromosomal inheritance, that are expressed in a codominant manner. The polymorphism of HLA genes in a non-inbred population is so great that there are no individuals with exactly the same set of MHC haplotypes, except for identical twins [30]. These individual variations could explain the different genetic susceptibility to develop GD [31]. Various alleles or combinations of alleles in HLA genes have been reported at the population level as either a risk or protective factor for GD with differences between ethnic groups.

In Caucasian populations, the HLA genes associated with increased risk of GD are HLA-DR3, DQB1*03:01, DQA1*05, DQB1*02, DQA1*0501, and DRB1*03, while the closely linked haplotypes DQA1*0201-DQB1*0302-

DRB1*07 or DQA1*0201-DQB1*02-DRB1*07 appears to be protective [1, 32].

In Asian populations, the alleles that conferred susceptibility to GD are DRB1*0803, DRB1*1602, DRB1*14:03, and DPB1*05:01, and the closely linked haplotypes DRB1*0803-DQB1*0601 and DRB1*1602-DQB1*0502. Patients with DRB1*1301-DQB1*0603 alleles developed GD at younger ages and were more frequently associated with larger goiter [1, 33-34].

The DRB1*0101, DRB1*0701, DRB1*1202, and DRB1*1302 alleles are weakly associated with resistance to developing GD. The DRB1*0701 allele confers a protective effect on GD in both Caucasian and Asian individuals [1, 33-34].

In African-American populations, the alleles DRB3*01:01, DRB3*02:02, and DQA1*05:01 associated with GD have been identified [35].

The expression of certain allelic polymorphisms in genes involved in the regulation of T cells can increase the risk of GD. Cytotoxic T-Lymphocyte Antigen 4 (CTLA-4) is an inhibitory receptor that down-regulate T cell activity. It is expressed on the membrane of T cells and due to its structural homology with the CD28 molecule, it is capable of binding B7 on antigen-presenting cells with greater affinity and avidity than CD28. Stimulation of the CTLA4 receptor reduces the adhesion time between the T cells and the antigen-presenting cell and, therefore, halts the activation of the T cells, decreasing the immune response [36]. The rs3087243 and rs231775 alleles of the CTLA4 gene were associated with an increased risk of GD in different ethnic groups. In addition, the rs231775 allelic polymorphism was more frequently associated with severe Graves' orbitopathy. Although the mechanisms are not known, it is postulated that defects in mRNA processing or post-translational glycosylation could alter its functionality [37]. These polymorphisms may act synergically with MHC polymorphisms such as HLA-DPB1*O5:01 [38]. An increased risk of GD has also been associated with the use of CTLA4-blocking drugs such as the monoclonal antibody ipilimumab directed against the receptor, used in the clinic for the treatment of some types of cancer, such as melanoma or small-cell lung cancer [39].

CD40 is expressed on antigen-presenting cells and acts as a co-regulator of T-cell activation, and contributes to B-cell activation and proliferation and to B-cell memory formation. The allelic variant rs1883832 was associated with an increased risk of GD in different ethnic groups [40].

CD25 (IL-2 receptor alpha subunit; IL-2Rα) encoded by the IL2RA/CD25 gene binds IL-2 that plays a pivotal role in the regulation of T cell function. Levels of a soluble form of IL-2Rα lacking the transmembrane and cytoplasmic domains were shown to be increased in patients with GD. The rs2104286, rs41295061, and rs11594656 allelic polymorphisms have been associated with increased concentrations of soluble IL-2Rα and greater susceptibility to GD [41].

The *FOXP3* gene is located on the X chromosome (Xp11.23) and encodes the Forkhead P3 protein (*FOXP3*), a transcription factor essential for the normal function of regulatory T cells, which play an important role in the prevention of autoimmunity. FOXP3 mutations induce IPEX syndrome in the male gender, which is lethal and includes immune dysregulation, polyendocrinopathy, and enteropathy [42]. The X chromosome location of *FOXP3* may contribute to the female predominance seen in GD. Meta-analysis studies have determined the association between the rs3761548, and rs3761549 single-nucleotide polymorphisms of the *FOXP3* gene and susceptibility to GD, subgroup analysis according to ethnicity showed that rs3761548 was associated with GD in Asians but not in Caucasians, whereas rs3761549 was associated in both Asians and Caucasians [43].

PTPN22 gene encodes a lymphocyte tyrosine phosphatase that inactivates the kinases associated with T-cell receptors, thus reducing T-cell activation. The rs2476601 polymorphisms have been associated with GD in Caucasian populations [44].

4.1.2. Thyroid-Specific Genes

GD is characterized by the presence of clones of T cells autoreactive against the TSH-R, for which main attention was paid to the study of gene polymorphisms that could be associated with GD. The polymorphisms that were associated with an increased risk of GD were rs179247, rs12101255, rs12101261, rs2268458, and rs12885526 in the Caucasian population [45]. It has been hypothesized that viral infections leading to the production of interferon-α could induce differential epigenetic changes in polymorphic regions, decreasing the expression of TSH-R in the thymus and the efficacy of negative selection of anti-TSH-R autoreactive T cell clones.

TG is a high molecular weight dimeric protein essential for the synthesis of thyroid hormones, and whose immunogenicity increases with the degree of iodination. The TGrl29 microsatellite in TG gene has been associated with an increased risk of GD [46]. The allelic variant W1999R (exon 33) of the TG gene when expressed with the HLA-DRB1*03 polymorphism increases the risk of GD [47]. A polymorphism in the promoter region of the TG gene at position -1623 increases transcription mediated by an interferon-inducible factor and is associated with an increased risk of GD, which supports the hypothesis of viral involvement in the pathogenesis of GD [48].

In fact, the genes that have been identified as predisposing to GD are only a minor part of the genetic contribution to the disease. Interestingly, the relatively low penetrance of GD in the case of genetic predisposition (twins or parents) suggests that endogenous and environmental factors are determinants for the development of the pathology.

4.2. Endogenous and Environmental Risk Factors

In addition to the genetic factors associated with GD, there are endogenous factors specific to the female gender that could explain its ten times higher prevalence with respect to men. The female predominance in GD suggests a crucial role played by estrogens in etiopathogenesis. Thus, a link has been reported between the level of estrogens and the expression of the B-cell activating factor (BAFF), an essential immunoregulator of autoimmune thyroid disease [49]. Higher expression of estrogen receptors has been described in thyroid tissue in patients with GD [50]. Otherwise, meta-analysis studies confirmed the importance of X-inactivation in the onset of GD in females [51]. Somatic cells have two X chromosomes in females, but only one is expressed since the other is randomly inactivated by methylation. Skewed X chromosome inactivation, arbitrarily defined by inactivation of the same X chromosome in 80% of cells is associated with GD, particularly in those patients unable to respond to antithyroid treatments [52].

Environmental factors also contribute to the onset of GD in genetically susceptible individuals, including infection by microorganisms, treatment with immunomodulatory drugs (such as those used in cancer therapies), endocrine disruptors, exposure to cigarette smoke and emotional stress conditions.

For years, the development of GD has been attributed to infectious processes caused by certain viruses and bacteria. Several authors have postulated cross-immunogenicity between bacterial and viral epitopes and thyroid antigens as a result of antigenic mimicry. This hypothesis gains strength after several reports demonstrated the presence of pathogen infections prior to the onset of GD. Thus, *Yersinia enterocolitica*, Coxsackie B, Retrovirus, *Helicobacter pylori*, and the hepatitis C virus have been associated with GD [53]. In this same sense, pregnancy would be another candidate because can trigger GD during the first weeks of gestation as a result of a cross-immune reaction between fetal antigens and maternal thyroid antigens.

In response to viral infections, different phenotype cells produce and secrete interferon (IFN), which is known to exert an immunomodulatory effect on the thyroid gland. Moreover, some reports indicate that the treatment with IFN-α in hepatitis C triggers thyroid autoimmunity in about 2% to 8% of patients, with an increased risk in female patients with ~~a~~ history of thyroid pathology [54]. An imbalance in the production of cytokines towards a proinflammatory profile has been found in patients with GD after infections with different pathogens, which could promote lymphocytic infiltration in the thyroid parenchyma activating the autoimmune response.

Several studies have demonstrated that cigarette smoking exerts multiple effects on the thyroid gland. Components in cigarette smoke increase serum thyroid hormone levels and decrease TSH levels. In addition, smoking has been identified as a risk factor for GD and particularly for Graves' orbitopathy. Smoking is related to the reduced effectiveness of antithyroid therapies followed by a higher recurrence rate of hyperthyroidism [55]. The risk of GD disappears sometime after smoking cessation, then is conceivable that its participation in thyroid autoimmunity could involve reversible epigenetic mechanisms. Therefore, it has been suggested that reactive oxygen species generated from cigarette smoking could alter epigenetic marks in immunomodulatory genes, contributing to the development and progression of GD [56].

Emotional stress definitely alters the immune function by inhibiting the cellular response and activating the humoral response. Some studies reported that stress is clinically diagnosed in 62-85% of GD patients. Indeed, a correlation has been found among the degree of emotional stress, serum levels of thyroid hormones and autoantibodies, and the intensity of symptoms [57].

Environmental or endogenous risk factors and genetic factors predisposing to GD could be linked through the induction of epigenetic mechanisms that result in reversible or irreversible epigenetic changes, such as DNA methylation, histone modification, or X chromosome inactivation. These epigenetic changes could induce the overexpression as well as the silencing of genes that are normally repressed or activated in euthyroid individuals, triggering thyroid autoimmunity.

Conclusion

GD is the most common source of hyperthyroidism, with a higher prevalence in the female gender, and can develop at any stage of life. However, the outbreak of the disease is more frequent between 30 and 60 years of age. Although it is admitted to have an autoimmune origin, the molecular mechanisms involved in the onset of the pathology have not been elucidated. For instance, different polymorphisms have been identified in immune and thyroid genes that confer genetic susceptibility to GD, but this is not enough for the development of the disease. Moreover, it has been recognized that the onset of GD is multifactorial, involving a complex interaction among endogenous, environmental, and genetic factors. Conventional antithyroid drug therapies restore thyroid hormone levels to euthyroid values, reducing symptoms of hyperthyroidism, but are not directed toward molecular targets involved in the immune response against thyroid self-antigens. Some patients require ablation of the thyroid by radioiodine or surgical thyroidectomy because they are unable to respond to antithyroid drugs or have disease remissions. The novel, more effective drugs against immune system targets, such as PDL-1 and CTLA-4, are under study in preclinical and clinical trials.

Knowledge of the etiopathogenic factors that may explain or contribute to the onset of GD provides opportunities to design new therapeutical approaches for autoimmune thyroid pathology.

References

[1] Wémeau, J. L., Klein, M., Sadoul, J. L., Briet, C., Vélayoudom-Céphise, F. L., (2018). Graves' disease: Introduction, epidemiology, endogenous and environmental pathogenic factors. *Ann Endocrinol.* 79(6), 599-607.

[2] Burch, H. B., Cooper, D. S., (2015). Management of Graves Disease: A Review. *JAMA* 314(23), 2544-2554.

[3] Smith, T. J., Hegedüs, L., (2016). Graves' Disease. *N Engl J Med.* 375(16), 1552-1565.

[4] Tsymbaliuk, I., Unukovych, D., Shvets, N., Dinets, A., (2015). Cardiovascular complications secondary to Graves' disease: a prospective study from Ukraine. *PLoS One* 10(3), e0122388.

[5] Bartley, G. B., Fatourechi, V., Kadrmas, E. F., Jacobsen, S. J., Ilstrup, D. M., Garrity, J. A., Gorman, C. A., (1996). Clinical features of Graves' ophthalmopathy in an incidence cohort. *Am J Ophthalmol.* 121 (3), 284-290.

[6] Hiromatsu, Y., Eguchi, H., Tani, J., Kasaoka, M., Teshima, Y., (2014). Graves' ophthalmopathy: epidemiology and natural history. *Intern Med.* 53(5), 353-360.

[7] Bunevicius, R., Prange, A. J., (2006). Psychiatric manifestations of Graves hyperthyroidism: pathophysiology and treatment options. *CNS Drugs* 20 (11), 897-909.

[8] Weetman, A. P., (2000). Graves' disease. *N Eng J Med.* 343(17), 1236-1248.

[9] Vanderpump, M. P. J., (2011). The epidemiology of thyroid disease. *Br Med Bull* 99, 39-51.

[10] Zimmermann, M. B., Boelaert, K., (2015). Iodine deficiency and thyroid disorders. *Lancet Diabetes Endocrinol.* 3(4), 286-295.

[11] Antonelli, A., Ferrari, S. M., Ragusa, F., Elia, G., Paparo, S. R., Ruffilli, I., Patrizio, A., Giusti, C., Gonnella, D., Cristaudo, A., Foddis, R., Shoenfeld, Y., Fallahi, P., (2020). Graves' disease: Epidemiology, genetic and environmental risk factors and viruses. *Best Pract Res Clin Endocrinol Metab.* 34(1), 101387.

[12] Mansourian, A. R., (2011). Metabolic pathways of tetraidothyronine and triidothyronine production by thyroid gland: a review of articles. *Pak J Biol Sci.* 14(1), 1-12.

[13] Karmisholt, J., Andersen, S., Laurberg, P., (2011). Variation in thyroid function in subclinical hypothyroidism: importance of clinical follow-up and therapy. *Eur J Endocrinol.* 164(3), 317-323.

[14] George, A., Diana, T., Längericht, J., Kahaly, G, J., (2021). Stimulatory thyrotropin receptor antibodies are a biomarker for Graves' Orbitopathy. *Front Endocrinol* 11:629925.

[15] Morshed, S. A., Davies, T. F., (2015). Graves' disease mechanisms: the role of stimulating, blocking, and cleavage region TSH receptor antibodies. *Horm Metab Res.* 47(10), 727-734.

[16] Lavard, L., Perrild, H., Jacobsen, B. B., Høier-Madsen, M., Bendinelli, G., Vitti, P., (2000). Prevalence of thyroid peroxidase, thyroglobulin and thyrotropin receptor antibodies in a long-term follow-up of juvenile Graves disease. *Autoimmunity* 32(3), 167-172.

[17] Marinò, M., Rotondo Dottore, G., Ionni, I., Lanzolla, G., Sabini, E., Ricci, D., Sframeli, A., Mazzi, B., Menconi, F., Latrofa, F., Vitti, P., Marcocci, C., Chiovato, L., (2019). Serum antibodies against the insulin-like growth factor-1 receptor (IGF-1R) in Graves' disease and Graves' orbitopathy. *J Endocrinol Invest.* 42(4), 471-480.

[18] Kocjan, T., Wraber, B., Repnik, U., Hojker, S., (2000). Changes in Th1/Th2 cytokine balance in Graves' disease. *Pflugers Arch.* 440(5 Suppl), R94-R95.

[19] Hesarghatta Shyamasunder, A., Abraham, P., (2017). Measuring TSH receptor antibody to influence treatment choices in Graves' disease. *Clin Endocrinol.* 86(5), 652-657.

[20] Kemp, E. H., Metcalfe, R. A., Smith, K. A., Woodroofe, M. N., Watson, P. F., Weetman A. P., (2003). Detection and localization of chemokine gene expression in autoimmune thyroid disease. *Clin Endocrinol* 59(2), 207-213.

[21] Matsunaga, M., Eguchi, K., Fukuda, T., Kurata, A., Tezuka, H., Shimomura, C., Otsubo, T., Ishikawa, N., Ito, K., Nagataki, S., (1986). Class II major histocompatibility complex antigen expression and cellular interactions in thyroid glands of Graves' disease. *J Clin Endocrinol Metab.* 62(4), 723-728.

[22] Faure, G. C., Bensoussan-Lejzerowicz, D., Bene, M. C., Aubert, V., Leclere, J., (1997). Coexpression of CD40 and class II antigen HLA-DR in Graves' disease thyroid epithelial cells. *Clin Immunol Immunopathol.* 84(2), 212-215.

[23] Hai, Y. P., Lee, A. C. H., Frommer, L., Diana, T., Kahaly, G. J., (2020). Immunohistochemical analysis of human orbital tissue in Graves' orbitopathy. *J Endocrinol Invest.* 43(2), 123-137.

[24] Wang, Y., Smith, T. J., (2014). Current concepts in the molecular pathogenesis of thyroid-associated ophthalmopathy. *Invest Ophthalmol Vis Sci.* 55(3), 1735-1748.

[25] Smith, T. J., Janssen, J. A. M. J. L., (2019). Insulin-like Growth Factor-I Receptor and Thyroid-Associated Ophthalmopathy. *Endocr Rev.* 40(1), 236-267.

[26] Krieger, C. C., Neumann, S., Gershengorn, M. C., (2020). TSH/IGF1 receptor crosstalk: Mechanism and clinical implications. *Pharmacol Ther.* 209, 107502.

[27] Łacheta, D., Miśkiewicz, P., Głuszko, A., Nowicka, G., Struga, M., Kantor, I., Poślednik, K. B., Mirza, S., Szczepański, M. J., (2019). Immunological Aspects of Graves' Ophthalmopathy. *Biomed Res Int.* 2019, 7453260.

[28] Draman, M. S., Zhang, L., Dayan, C., Ludgate, M. M (2021). Orbital Signaling in Graves' Orbitopathy. *Front Endocrinol.* 12, 739994.

[29] Kahaly, G. J., (2020). Management of Graves Thyroidal and Extrathyroidal Disease: An Update. *J Clin Endocrinol Metab.* 105(12), 3704-3720.

[30] Rask, L., Jonsson, A. K., Svensson, A. C., Gustafsson, K., Andersson, L., (1991). The structure of human MHC class II genes. *Autoimmunity* 8(3), 237-244.

[31] Hunt, P. J., Marshall, S. E., Weetman, A. P., Bunce, M., Bell, J. I., Wass, J. A., Welsh, K. I., (2001). Histocompatibility leucocyte antigens and closely linked immunomodulatory genes in autoimmune thyroid disease. *Clin Endocrinol* 55(4), 491-499.

[32] Yanagawa, T., Mangklabruks, A., Chang, Y. B., Okamoto, Y., Fisfalen, M. E., Curran, P. G., DeGroot, L. J., (1993). Human histocompatibility leukocyte antigen-DQA1*0501 allele associated with genetic susceptibility to Graves' disease in a Caucasian population. *J Clin Endocrinol Metab.* 76(6), 1569-1574.

[33] Park, M. H., Park, Y. J., Song, E. Y., Park, H., Kim, T. Y., Park, D. J., Park, K. S., Cho, B. Y., (2005). Association of HLA-DR and -DQ genes with Graves disease in Koreans. *Hum Immunol.* 66(6), 741-747.

[34] Okada, Y., Momozawa, Y., Ashikawa, K., Kanai, M., Matsuda, K., Kamatani, Y., Takahashi, A., Kubo, M., (2015). Construction of a population-specific HLA imputation reference panel and its application to Graves' disease risk in Japanese. *Nat Genet.* 47(7), 798-802.

[35] Chen, Q. Y., Nadell, D., Zhang, X. Y., Kukreja, A., Huang, Y. J., Wise, J., Svec, F., Richards, R., Friday, K. E., Vargas, A., Gomez, R., Chalew, S., Lan, M. S., Tomer, Y., Maclaren, N. K. (2000). The human leukocyte antigen HLA DRB3*020/DQA1*0501 haplotype is associated with Graves' disease in African Americans. *J Clin Endocrinol Metab.* 85(4), 1545-1549.

[36] Kosmaczewska, A., Ciszak, L., Boćko, D., Frydecka, I., (2001). Expression and functional significance of CTLA-4, a negative regulator of T cell activation. *Arch Immunol Ther Exp.* 49(1), 39-46.

[37] Tu, Y., Fan, G., Dai, Y., Zeng, T., Xiao F., Chen, L., Kong, W., (2017). Association between rs3087243 and rs231775 polymorphism within the cytotoxic T-lymphocyte antigen 4 gene and Graves' disease: a case/control study combined with meta-analyses. *Oncotarget* 8(66), 110614-110624.

[38] Simmonds, M. J., Gough, S. C., (2004). Unravelling the genetic complexity of autoimmune thyroid disease: HLA, CTLA-4 and beyond. *Clin Exp Immunol.* 136(1), 1-10.

[39] Borodic, G., Hinkle, D. M., Cia, Y. (2011). Drug-induced graves disease from CTLA-4 receptor suppression. *Ophthalmic Plast Reconstr Surg.* 27(4), e87-e88.

[40] Wang, X. X., Wang, X. X., Chen, T., (2019). Association between the CD40 rs1883832 polymorphism and Graves' disease risk: a meta-analysis. *EXCLI J.* 18, 10-20.

[41] Chistiakov, D. A., Chistiakova, E. I., Voronova, N. V., Turakulov, R. I., Savost'anov, K. V., (2011). A variant of the Il2ra / Cd25 gene predisposing to graves' disease is associated with increased levels of soluble interleukin-2 receptor. *Scand J Immunol.* 74(5), 496-501.

[42] Huang, Q., Liu, X., Zhang, Y., Huang, J., Li, D., Li, B., (2020). Molecular feature and therapeutic perspectives of immune dysregulation, polyendocrinopathy, enteropathy, X-linked syndrome. *J Genet Genomics* 47(1), 17-26.

[43] Tan, G., Wang, X., Zheng, G., Du, J., Zhou, F., Liang, Z., Wei, W., Yu. H., (2021). Meta-analysis reveals significant association between FOXP3 polymorphisms and susceptibility to Graves' disease. *J Int Med Res.* 49(4), 3000605211004199.

[44] Heward, J. M., Brand, O. J., Barrett, J. C., Carr-Smith, J. D., Franklyn, J. A., Gough, S. C., (2007). Association of PTPN22 haplotypes with Graves' disease. *J Clin Endocrinol Metab.* 92(2), 685-690.

[45] Xiong, H., Wu, M., Yi, H., Wang, X., Wang, Q., Nadirshina, S., Zhou, X., Liu, X., (2016). Genetic associations of the thyroid stimulating hormone receptor gene with Graves diseases and Graves ophthalmopathy: A meta-analysis. *Sci Rep.* 6, 30356.

[46] Caputo, M., Rivolta, C. M., Mories, T., Corrales, J. J., Galindo, P., González-Sarmiento, R., Targovnik, H. M., Miralles-García, J. M., (2010). Analysis of thyroglobulin gene polymorphisms in patients with autoimmune thyroiditis. *Endocrine* 37(3), 389-395.

[47] Ban, Y., Greenberg, D. A., Concepcion, E., Skrabanek, L., Villanueva, R., Tomer, Y., (2003). Amino acid substitutions in the thyroglobulin gene are associated with susceptibility to human and murine autoimmune thyroid disease. *Proc Natl Acad Sci.* 100(25), 15119-15124.

[48] Stefan M., Jacobson, E. M., Huber, A. K., Greenberg, D. A., Li, C. W., Skrabanek, L., Conception, E., Fadlalla, M., Ho, K., Tomer, Y., (2011). Novel variant of thyroglobulin promoter triggers thyroid autoimmunity through an epigenetic interferon alpha-modulated mechanism. *J Biol Chem.* 286(36), 31168-31179.

[49] Cheng, C. W., Fang, W. F., Tang, K. T., Lin, J. D., (2021). Possible interplay between estrogen and the BAFF may modify thyroid activity in Graves' disease. *Sci Rep.* 11(1), 21350.

[50] Domoslawski, P., Podhorska-Okolow, M., Pula, B., Lukienczuk, T., Dziegiel, P., (2013). Expression of estrogen and progesterone receptors and Ki-67 antigen in Graves' disease and nodular goiter. *Folia Histochem Cytobiol.* 51(2), 135-140.

[51] Simmonds, M. J., Kavvoura, F. K., Brand, O. J., Newby, P. R., Jackson, L. E., Hargreaves, C. E., Franklyn, J. A., Gough, S. C. L., (2014). Skewed X chromosome inactivation and female preponderance in autoimmune thyroid disease: an association study and meta-analysis. *J Clin Endocrinol Metab.* 99(1), E127-E131.

[52] Ishido, N., Inoue, N., Watanabe, M., Hidaka, Y., Iwatani, Y., (2015). The relationship between skewed X chromosome inactivation and the prognosis of Graves' and Hashimoto's diseases. Thyroid 25(2), 256-261.

[53] Valtonen, V. V., Ruutu, P., Varis, K., Ranki, M., Malkamäki, M., Mäkelä, P. H., (1986). Serological evidence for the role of bacterial infections in the pathogenesis of thyroid diseases. *Acta Med Scand.* 219(1), 105-111.

[54] Maiga, I., Valdes-Socin, H., Thiry, A., Delwaide, J., Sidibe, A. T., Beckers, A., (2015). Alpha interferon induced hyperthyroidism: a case report and review of the literature]. *Rev Med Liege* 70(7-8), 390-394.

[55] Wiersinga, W. M., (2013). Smoking and thyroid. *Clin Endocrinol.* 79(2), 145-151.

[56] Sabana, M., Costilla, M., Klecha, A. J., Di Cugno, M., Curria, M. I., Cremaschi, G., Barreiro Arcos, M. L., (2021). Regulation of the cellular redox state and the expression of DNA methyltransferase-1 in peripheral blood mononuclear cells from patients with Graves' disease. *Endocr Diab Nutr.* doi:10.1016/j.endinu.2021.07.011e Graves.

[57] Falgarone, G., Heshmati, H. M., Cohen, R., Reach, G., (2012). Mechanisms in endocrinology. Role of emotional stress in the pathophysiology of Graves' disease. *Eur J Endocrinol.* 168(1), R13-R18.

Chapter 3

The Epidemiology and Pathophysiology of Toxic Multinodular Goiter, Toxic Thyroid Adenoma, and Other Autonomous Causes of Hyperthyroidism

Prathosh Gangadhar*, MD, DM

Department of Endocrinology, IQRAA Hospital and Research Centre, Kozhikode, Kerala, India

Abstract

This chapter will discuss the epidemiological and pathophysiologic aspects of autonomous causes of hyperthyroidism. The most common autonomous causes of hyperthyroidism include Toxic multinodular goiter (TMNG) and toxic thyroid adenoma (TA). Both are associated with somatic mutations of the TSH receptor. Rarely germ line TSH receptor activating mutations produce inherited non-autoimmune hyperthyroidism. Somatic mutations of the TSH receptors and Gs α protein are responsible for functional autonomy of the Thyroid in 20-80% of cases. Thus, many nodules have an undetermined cause of functional autonomy. Iodine deficiency contributes higher incidence of these mutations. Non-functioning nodules in the same gland lack these mutations. Second hit EZH1 gene mutations were detected in 27% of cases of TAs. This leads to thyrocyte proliferation and growth factor expression resulting in the development of small clones which further form foci leading to nodule formation. The advantageous mutation leads

* Corresponding Author's Email: prathosh@yahoo.com.

In: Understanding and Managing Hyperthyroidism
Editor: Poongkodi Karunakaran
ISBN: 979-8-88697-636-6

to function and proliferation (TSHR mutations) or proliferation (RAS mutations) alone determines nodules' final functional status.

Keywords: toxic multinodular goiter, toxic thyroid adenoma, autonomously functioning thyroid nodule, inherited non-autoimmune hyperthyroidism, thyroid autonomy, mutagenesis, TSH receptor mutations, iodine deficiency

1. Introduction

Thyroid autonomy manifests as toxic adenoma and toxic multinodular goiter. Thyroid autonomy is a condition where Thyrocytes function and produce thyroid hormones independently of TSH and without TSH receptor stimulating antibodies. This increase in the secretion of thyroid hormones leads to suppression of TSH and proliferation of the unaffected thyroid tissue [1].

1.1. Diagnosis of Thyroid Autonomy

Clinically, thyroid autonomy presents with features of thyrotoxicosis and is generally associated with thyroid nodules. Many autonomous nodules will show only subclinical thyroid dysfunction. Constitutive activation of TSH receptor (TSHR) or, less frequently, the alpha subunit of G protein by somatic mutations in their respective genes have been identified as the predominant molecular cause of thyroid autonomy. TA is a solitary Autonomously Functioning Thyroid Nodule (AFTN) leading to thyrotoxicosis. TMNG is a heterogeneous clinical disorder characterized by the presence of goiter with a hyperfunctioning single hot nodule or hot nodules with or without additional nodules with normal or decreased uptake on scintigraphy. TMNG comprises the most frequent form of thyroid autonomy. Very rarely, autosomal dominantly inherited non-autoimmune hyperthyroidism caused by activating germline mutations in the TSH receptor gene can present with thyroid autonomy. Clinical features include the presence of thyrotoxicosis and goiter in at least two generations with negative workup for Graves' disease. This condition will recur in all patients after withdrawal of anti-thyroid treatment or partial thyroidectomy. Inherited non-autoimmune hyperthyroidism should be suspected in case of neonatal thyrotoxicosis and unusually relapsing non-autoimmune thyrotoxicosis in childhood, even if there is no family history [2], [3].

2. Epidemiology

Thyroid autonomy is a common finding in iodine deficiency areas where it accounts for up to 60 percent of cases (TA - about 10%, TMNG - about 50%) [4]. Euthyroid MNG to TMNG transition develops insidiously. The most accurate epidemiological data showed that toxic adenoma natural course is slow. In a group of 375 untreated euthyroid patients with TA in Germany, who were followed for a mean period of 53 months, the annual incidence of thyrotoxicosis was 4.1% [5]. In two longitudinal studies, 9-10% of overt thyrotoxicosis has been reported in patients with euthyroid MNG over a mean follow-up period of up to 12.2 years [6, 7]. Nodule size correlates with the development of hyperthyroidism: In a US study, 93.5% of patients with overt hyperthyroidism had TA greater than 3 cm in the greatest dimension. TA of greater than 3 cm in the greatest dimension and euthyroid during presentation carried a 20% risk of developing hyperthyroidism during a 6-year follow-up period as opposed to a 2-5% risk in patients with nodules less than 2.5 cm in the greatest dimension [8].

3. Pathophysiology

Benign thyroid nodules can be hyperplastic nodules (adenomatous nodules) - nodules without a capsule and true nodule - with a definite fibrous capsule. Often distinction will be difficult between these nodules, especially with co-existing thyroiditis and goiter. Nodules based on scintigraphy appearance can be classified as normal, cold, and hot, which denotes the functional status of nodules [9, 10].

In contrast to solitary nodular thyroid disease, which has a more uniform clinical, pathological, and molecular picture, euthyroid multinodular goiter (MNG) and toxic multinodular goiter (TMNG) are a mixed group of nodular entities, i.e., one usually finds a combination of hyper-functional, hypofunctional, or normally functioning thyroid lesions within the same thyroid gland. The overall balance of functional properties of individual thyroid nodules within a multinodular goiter ultimately determines the functional status of the individual patient, which may be euthyroidism (normal

TSH and free thyroid hormone levels), subclinical hyperthyroidism (low or suppressed TSH and normal free thyroid hormone levels), or overt hyperthyroidism (suppressed TSH and elevated free thyroid hormone levels). The term MNG is applied to the first scenario, whereas TMNG refers to the latter situation. Only 10% of autonomously functioning nodules show clinical thyrotoxicosis. Therefore, a suppression scan can be performed on a euthyroid person with suspected autonomy. Levothyroxine 75 mcg/day for two weeks, followed by 150 mcg/day for the next two weeks, supplemented to suppress non -autonomous thyroid tissue uptake and help to unmask thyroid autonomy [11].

It is important to emphasize that this functional picture is not stationary, but patients with TMNG usually have a history of long-standing MNG. Moreover, the status of TSH suppression in TMNG does not only imply clinical consequences for the patient but, importantly, it also indicates a critical level of thyroid autonomy, i.e., independence of TSH, the physiological regulator of thyroid function and growth, has been reached [10].

3.1. Hyperplastic Growth to Nodular Transformation

The starting point of all TMNG or TA is hyperplasia induced by iodine deficiency. Iodine deficiency is the key exogenous factor. Other factors include goitrogens, pregnancy, smoking, and selenium deficiency. Iodine deficiency increases mutagenesis directly (production of H_2O_2/free radicals) [12] or indirectly (Thyrocyte proliferation and increased number of cell divisions). Further hyperplasia leads to the formation of cell clones; some carry somatic mutations of TSHR leading to TA or contain mutations that lead to dedifferentiation and, therefore, cold thyroid nodules. Mutations in the genes encoding the TSH receptor (TSHR) or the Gs protein α subunit (Gs α) are found in approximately 70% of TA s. The thyroid gland undergoes hyperplasia, and the expression of growth factors (e.g., IGF-I, EGF) is increased [9]. Due to this growth factor co-stimulation, most cells divide and form small clones. Inactivation of TGF-β1 signaling in TAs due to constitutively activated TSHR pathway leads not only to thyrocyte proliferation but also to inhibition of iodine uptake, iodine organification, and thyroglobulin expression [13]. After growth factor expression, small clones with activating mutations will further proliferate. They form small foci which develop into thyroid nodules. This mechanism explains hot nodules by advantageous mutations which initiate both growth and function of affected thyroid cells. Cold nodules develop by a mutation that stimulates proliferation only (e.g., RAS mutations). In the subset of patients with normal thyroid function and thyroid nodules, the growth of thyroid nodules may be a local process not associated with the growth of the surrounding non-nodular tissue. In such a situation, it should be referred to more appropriately as uni-or multinodular 'thyroid gland' instead of 'goiter' [14].

In some subset of individuals, when they are exposed to iodine deficiency, they do not develop a goiter. The mechanism of this adaptation is poorly understood, but data from the mouse model suggest an increase in mRNA expression of TSH receptor, NIS, and TPO in response to iodine deficiency which is a sign of increased iodine turnover in thyroid cells [15].

3.2. What Drives Thyroid Autonomy - The Transformation to Hot Thyroid Nodules?

In 1989, Dumont et al. suggested that overactivity of the cAMP system could account for benign thyroid tumors and that molecular defects resulting in signaling through the cAMP cascade might be responsible for the autonomous function of thyroid epithelial cells. This reasoning came from identifying somatic mutations in the Gs α protein that lead to constitutive activation of the cAMP cascade resulting in GH-producing pituitary adenomas [16]. However, these mutations provided a molecular explanation for a limited number of benign thyroid tumors. Therefore, signaling proteins other than Gs α had to be considered [17].

Constitutive activation of the cAMP signaling pathway is widely accepted as the biochemical driving force of thyroid autonomy, as suggested by the presence of somatic activating TSH receptor (TSHR) mutations in scintigraphically non-suppressible foci in euthyroid goiters in iodine-deficient areas; the presence of somatic TSHR mutations (80%) and, less frequently, Gs α protein mutations (4%) in macroscopic toxic thyroid nodules both in solitary nodules and multinodular disease. Parma and co-workers identified TSHR mutations in hyperfunctioning thyroid nodules.

The involvement of other genes and the pathogenesis of the remaining cases are presently unknown. Whole-exome sequencing in 19 TAs identified a recurrent hot-spot mutation (c. 1712A > G; p. Gln571Arg) in the enhancer of zeste homolog 1 (EZH1) gene, which codes for a catalytic subunit of the polycomb complex. This mutation occurs with high frequency (27%) in TAs. EZH1 mutations are strongly associated with known (TSHR, Gs α) or alterations in cAMP pathway genes. EZH1 mutation causes increased histone H3 trimethylation and increases the proliferation of thyroid cells. This hot-spot mutation in EZH1 is the second most frequent genetic alteration in TAs. The association between EZH1 and TSHR mutations proposes a 2-hit model for tumor pathogenesis [18].

Henceforth, constitutive activation of the cAMP pathway and EZH1 mutations cooperate to induce the hyperproliferation of thyroid cells.

3.3. Is Thyroid Autonomy Synonymous with Benign Thyroid Disease?

In the past, thyroid autonomy is widely viewed as an exclusively benign disease. However, more than 60 case reports of thyroid carcinoma within a hot nodule have been published. The incidence of toxic thyroid cancer varied from 0.7% to 6% in different series [14]. A recent study showed a malignancy rate of 8.5% in combined hyperthyroid and euthyroid hot nodules [19]. Further animal data suggested the development of large papillary thyroid cancer in nearly all mice with constitutively activating thyroid TSH receptor mutations, which is the most common etiology of hot nodules and rare inherited non-autoimmune hyperthyroidism. Twenty-one cases of somatic TSH receptor mutations positive hyperfunctioning thyroid carcinomas have been reported in the literature [20], and there is a dearth of data regarding the malignancy risk of hot nodules.

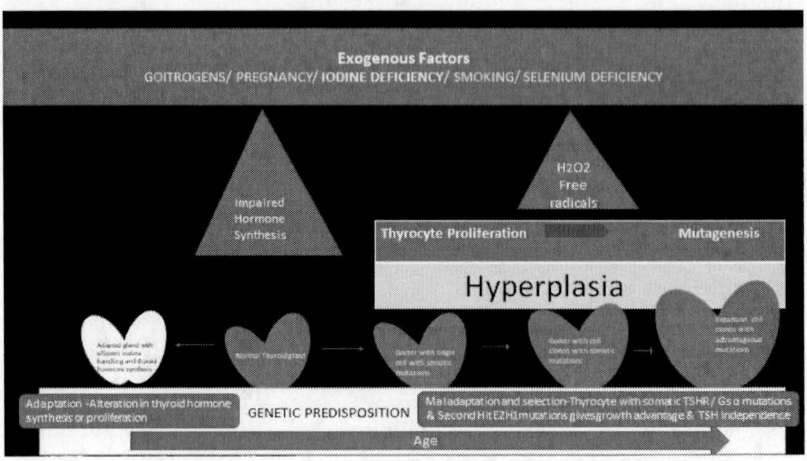

Figure 1. Pathophysiology of thyroid autonomy in a nutshell.

Conclusion

Autonomous causes of hyperthyroidism are TMNG, TA, and Inherited non-autoimmune hyperthyroidism due to germline TSHR mutations. Unlike TA, the overall balance of functional–status of thyroid nodules within an MNG determines its functionality. A patient with euthyroid MNG can have an autonomous nodule which can be revealed with a suppression scan. Iodine deficiency is the most common external factor that triggers Thyrocyte hyperplasia. Some thyroid gland adapts to iodine deficiency by altering thyroid hormone synthesis and cell proliferation. Iodine deficiency increases mutagenesis through H_2O_2 and free radicals, this leads to cell clones that carry somatic mutations. TSHR mutations trigger thyroid autonomy in many nodules. Gsα mutations contribute to a very small percentage of autonomous nodules. The second hit with a novel EZH1 mutation leads to thyroid autonomy in around 27% of TAs with TSHR mutations. Unlike the previous notion, thyroid autonomy is not synonymous with benign thyroid disease. TSHR mutation-positive hot thyroid carcinomas are increasingly reported in the literature, opening a new Pandora's box.

References

[1] K. Krohn and R. Paschke, "Progress in Understanding the Etiology of Thyroid Autonomy 1," *J. Clin. Endocrinol. Metab.*, vol. 86, no. 7, pp. 3336-3345, Jul. 2001, doi: 10.1210/jcem.86.7.7642.

[2] C. Ferraz and R. Paschke, "Inheritable and sporadic non-autoimmune hyperthyroidism," *Best Pract. Res. Clin. Endocrinol. Metab.*, vol. 31, no. 2, pp. 265-275, 2017, doi: 10.1016/j.beem.2017.04.005.

[3] S. Kosugi, "Non-autoimmune hyperthyroidism and hyperfunctioning thyroid adenomas caused by activating mutation of the thyrotropin receptor," *Nihon Rinsho.*, vol. 60, no. 2, pp. 291-6, Feb. 2002 [Online]. Available: http://www.ncbi.nlm.nih.gov/pubmed/11857916.

[4] P. Laurberg, K. M. Pedersen, H. Vestergaard, and G. Sigurdsson, "High incidence of multinodular toxic goiter in the elderly population in a low iodine intake area vs. high incidence of Graves' disease in the young in a high iodine intake area: comparative surveys of thyrotoxicosis epidemiology in East-Jutland Denmark a," *J. Intern. Med.*, vol. 229, no. 5, pp. 415-20, May 1991, doi: 10.1111/j.1365-2796.1991.tb00368.x.

[5] D. Sandrock, T. Olbricht, D. Emrich, G. Benker, and D. Reinwein, "Long-term follow-up in patients with autonomous thyroid adenoma," *Acta Endocrinol. (Copenh).*, vol. 128, no. 1, pp. 51-5, Jan. 1993, doi: 10.1530/acta.0.1280051.

[6] J. W. Elite, J. K. Bussemaker, and A. Haak, "The natural history of euthyroid multinodular goiter," *Postgrad. Med. J.*, vol. 66, no. 773, pp. 186-190, Mar. 1990, doi: 10.1136/pgmj.66.773.186.

[7] J. D. Wiener and A. A. de Vries, "On the natural history of Plummer's disease," *Clin. Nucl. Med.*, vol. 4, no. 5, pp. 181-90, May 1979, doi: 10.1097/00003072-197905000-00002.

[8] J. I. Hamburger, "Evolution of Toxicity in Solitary Nontoxic Autonomously Functioning Thyroid Nodules," *J. Clin. Endocrinol. Metab.*, vol. 50, no. 6, pp. 1089-1093, Jun. 1980, doi: 10.1210/jcem-50-6-1089.

[9] K. Krohn, D. Führer, Y. Bayer, M. Eszlinger, V. Brauer, S. Neumann, R. Paschke, D. Führer-Sakel, "Molecular pathogenesis of euthyroid and toxic multinodular goiter," *Endocr. Rev.*, vol. 26, no. 4, pp. 504-24, Jun. 2005, doi: 10.1210/er.2004-0005.

[10] M. Tonacchera and D. Führer, "Toxic Adenoma and Multinodular Toxic Goiter," 2018, pp. 513-539.

[11] M. Bähre, R. Hilgers, C. Lindemann, and D. Emrich, "Thyroid autonomy: sensitive detection in vivo and estimation of its functional relevance using quantified high-resolution scintigraphy," *Acta Endocrinol. (Copenh).*, vol. 117, no. 2, pp. 145-153, Feb. 1988, doi: 10.1530/acta.0.1170145.

[12] K. Krohn, J. Maier, and R. Paschke, "Mechanisms of disease: hydrogen peroxide, DNA damage and mutagenesis in the development of thyroid tumors," *Nat. Clin. Pract. Endocrinol. Metab.*, vol. 3, no. 10, pp. 713-20, Oct. 2007, doi: 10.1038/ncpendmet0621.

[13] M. Taton, F. Lamy, P. P. Roger, and J. E. Dumont, "General inhibition by transforming growth factor-beta 1 of thyrotropin and cAMP responses in human thyroid cells in primary culture," *Mol. Cell. Endocrinol.*, vol. 95, no. 1-2, pp. 13-21, Sep. 1993, doi: 10.1016/0303-7207(93)90024-e.

[14] R. Paschke, "*Toxic Adenoma and Toxic Multinodular Goiter" in The Thyroid*, 11th edit. Philadelphia: Wolters Kluwer, 2020.

[15] J. E. Dumont, A. M. Ermans, C. Maenhaut, F. Coppée, and J. B. Stanbury, "Large goitre as a maladaptation to iodine deficiency," *Clin. Endocrinol. (Oxf).*, vol. 43, no. 1, pp. 1-10, Jul. 1995, doi: 10.1111/j.1365-2265.1995.tb01886.x.

[16] J. E. Dumont, J. C. Jauniaux, and P. P. Roger, "The cyclic AMP-mediated stimulation of cell proliferation," *Trends Biochem. Sci.*, vol. 14, no. 2, pp. 67-71, Feb. 1989, doi: 10.1016/0968-0004(89)90046-7.

[17] J. Parma, L. Duprez, J. Van Sande, P. Cochaux, C. Gervy, J. Mockel, J. Dumont, and G. Vassart, "Somatic mutations in the thyrotropin receptor gene cause hyperfunctioning thyroid adenomas," *Nature*, vol. 365, no. 6447, pp. 649-51, Oct. 1993, doi: 10.1038/365649a0.

[18] D. Calebiro, E. Grassi, M. Eszlinger, C. Ronchi, A. Godbole, K. Bathon, F. Guizzardi, T. de Filippis, K. Krohn, H. Jaeschke, T. Schwarzmayr, R. Bircan, H. I. Gozu, S. Sancak, M. Niedziela, T. M. Strom, M. Fassnacht, L. Persani, and R. Paschke, "Recurrent EZH1 mutations are a second hit in autonomous thyroid adenomas," *J. Clin. Invest.*, vol. 126, no. 9, pp. 3383-8, 2016, doi: 10.1172/JCI84894.

[19] A. Dirikoc, S. B. Polat, Z. Kandemir, C. Aydin, D. Ozdemir, F. D. Dellal, R. Ersoy,and B. Cakir, "Comparison of ultrasonography features and malignancy rate of toxic and nontoxic autonomous nodules: a preliminary study," *Ann. Nucl. Med.*, vol. 29, no. 10, pp. 883-9, Dec. 2015, doi: 10.1007/s12149-015-1018-y.

[20] R. Paschke, "Thyroid Stimulating Hormone Receptor (TSHR) Mutation Database, Accessed on June 2022." https://tsh-receptor-mutationdatabase.org/prevalence.html.

Chapter 4

Organ System Manifestations of Hyperthyroidism

Nikitha Sriramaneni[1,*], MD
and Chitra Selvan[2,†], MD, DM
Department of Endocrinology, M.S. Ramaiah Medical College and Hospital, Bangalore, Karnataka

Abstract

The clinical spectrum of manifestations of hyperthyroidism ranges widely and depends on factors like age of onset, duration, and severity of hyperthyroidism etc. Neuromuscular manifestations include tremors, chorea, and myopathy. Thyrotoxic periodic paralysis and myasthenia gravis are rare. Common Neuropsychiatric manifestations include restlessness, irritability, anxiety, depression, and emotional lability. Infrequently, hyperthyroidism can present as encephalopathy, psychosis, and coma. Cardiovascular manifestations could be life-threatening like ischemia, atrial fibrillation, and heart failure. Takotsubo cardiomyopathy can be associated. Dyspnea on exertion and worsening of chronic lung disorders are common pulmonary manifestations. There is an increased frequency of bowel movements and steatorrhea due to fat malabsorption. Hepatic dysfunction can occur in severe cases. Celiac disease, pernicious anemia, and autoimmune hepatitis can coexist. Eyelid retraction and lid lag are commonly seen. Skin changes include flushing, increased diaphoresis, and palmar erythema. Onycholysis is characteristic but uncommon. Hair is fine and friable and there is increased hair loss.

* Corresponding Author's Email: snikitha3@gmail.com.
† Corresponding Author's Email: drchitraselvan@gmail.com.

In: Understanding and Managing Hyperthyroidism
Editor: Poongkodi Karunakaran
ISBN: 979-8-88697-636-6

Vitiligo is commonly associated. Renal blood flow and glomerular filtration is increased. Advanced cases can manifest as muscle wasting, and fractures due to net demineralization of bone. Hematologic manifestations include normocytic normochromic anemia, relative neutropenia, and lymphocytosis. Hypercoagulability is common due to enhanced factor VIII activity. Reproductive function is impaired.

Keywords: hyperthyroidism, Graves' disease, thyrotoxicosis, tachycardia, Graves' orbitopathy, hypertension

1. Introduction

The clinical manifestations of hyperthyroidism vary and are independent of its cause. Graves' disease, the most common cause of hyperthyroidism, can cause unique manifestations such as Graves' orbitopathy and infiltrative dermopathy in addition to other manifestations of hyperthyroidism. Most patients with hyperthyroidism present with a constellation of symptoms. This chapter enumerates the various organ system manifestations of hyperthyroidism.

2. Cardiovascular System

Most of the effects of thyroid hormones on the heart are mediated through triiodothyronine (T3). T3 increases the force and speed of systolic contraction and the speed of diastolic relaxation [1]. T3 decreases vascular resistance, including coronary vascular tone, and increases coronary arteriolar angiogenesis [1]. Thyroid hormones lead to reduced vascular tone and maintenance of normal arteriolar remodeling [1]. Triiodothyronine promotes vascular smooth muscle relaxation [1].

The clinical presentation of hyperthyroidism includes systolic hypertension, systolic murmurs, increased left ventricular mass, exercise intolerance, and angina pectoris [2]. Complications include atrial fibrillation with its risk of stroke and high output heart failure [3]. Atrial fibrillation can cause heart failure in the presence of pre-existent heart disease. The loss of atrial contractile function and decreased diastolic filling time due to tachycardia may cause increased filling pressures, contributing to cardiomyopathy.

While sinus tachycardia is the most common arrhythmia seen in hyperthyroidism, the incidence of atrial fibrillation ranges from 2% to 20% [4]. Hypertrophy, usually increased left ventricular mass, results from sustained volume overload and the resulting increase in cardiac work [5]. Pulmonary artery pressure is increased in hyperthyroidism which in turn can lead to right heart failure. Cardiovascular manifestations of hyperthyroidism can potentially cause life-threatening consequences.

3. Kidney

Thyroid hormone stimulates the renin-angiotensin system in several ways, including the increase in renin gene expression, synthesis of angiotensinogen by the liver, and plasma renin, angiotensin II and angiotensin converting enzyme levels [6]. This might lead to an increase in blood pressure. Hyperthyroidism increases renal blood flow and GFR. Activation of the renin-angiotensin system and the decrease in the resistance of afferent glomerular arterioles leads to an increase in the glomerular hydrostatic pressure and GFR [7].

The increase in GFR and the decrease in overall muscle mass lead to a reduction in serum creatinine levels. Serum cystatin C levels are elevated. Hyperthyroidism can cause polyuria due to direct downregulation of aquaporin channels along with increased blood pressure, cardiac output, and renal blood flow [8]. Hyperthyroidism is associated with a decreased ability to concentrate urine, a decrease in total body water, and exchangeable potassium [9]. Therapy of thyrotoxicosis can lead to normalization of renal function [10].

4. Neuropsychiatric

In elderly people, hyperthyroidism can cause agitation and apathy [11]. In some observational studies, subclinical hyperthyroidism was found to be associated with alterations in cognitive function [12]. Other manifestations of hyperthyroidism include restlessness, irritability, emotional lability, anxiety, depression, mania, delusional behavior, hallucinations, and dementia. Psychosis, encephalopathy, and coma are infrequent.

5. Central Nervous System

Seizures are only seen in a minority of patients (<1%) with moderate thyrotoxicosis. Thyroid storm can rarely present as febrile seizures in children [13]. Embolic and ischemic cerebrovascular events have been described in patients with overt thyrotoxicosis.

Visual disturbances in thyrotoxicosis occur primarily as a complication of Graves orbitopathy due to optic nerve compression at the apex of the orbit, diplopia related to extraocular muscle dysfunction, or, rarely, damage to the cornea. Sensorineural hearing loss, while common in hypothyroidism, rarely occurs in thyrotoxicosis, and has been attributed to an adverse drug effect of thionamides [14]. Impaired sensation resulting from peripheral neuropathy can occur in thyrotoxicosis [15]. An altered sense of smell can occur as a complication of orbital decompression surgery in patients with Graves orbitopathy. Disorders of taste can occur in hyperthyroidism.

Tremor associated with thyrotoxicosis is most evident in the hands but can occur in the tongue, trunk, and lower extremities. Chorea has been described in thyrotoxic patients and resolves following successful treatment of the patient's thyroid condition [16]. Myopathy, frequently proximal in location, occurs in the majority of patients with overt thyrotoxicosis. Myasthenia gravis occurs in less than 1% of patients with Graves' disease [17]. Thyrotoxic periodic paralysis results from an intracellular shift of potassium in a genetically and clinically susceptible patient. Sporadic paroxysmal kinesigenic dyskinesia (PKD) secondary to thyrotoxicosis is an extremely rare entity [18]. It is perhaps a result of a metabolic disturbance of the basal ganglia circuits rather than a permanent and irreversible change [18].

6. Gastrointestinal System

Hyperthyroidism is accompanied by normal gastric emptying with low acid production, partly due to autoimmune gastritis with hypergastrinemia [19]. Diarrhea is due to an accelerated transit time in the gut. Hyperphagia and adrenergic stimulations cause steatorrhea. Autoimmune gastritis and celiac disease are frequently associated with Graves' disease [20]. Thyrotoxicosis may present with gastrointestinal symptoms in the presence of coexisting adrenal pathology due to accelerated cortisol metabolism [21].

Hepatic changes with thyroid hormone excess typically consist of mild elevations in serum transaminases levels. Mild transaminase elevation can occur in the first few months of treatment with propylthiouracil in thyrotoxic patients, but this resolves with continued therapy. In severe thyrotoxicosis, associated cardiac failure can cause hepatic congestion leading to jaundice. Rarely autoimmune hepatitis can coexist with graves hyperthyroidism [22].

7. Respiratory System

Dyspnea on exertion is common in thyrotoxicosis. Contributing factors include respiratory muscle weakness [23], enhanced ventilatory drive, diminished lung compliance, and heart failure. Vital capacity is reduced.

Immunoglobulin E (IgE) levels are elevated in 30% of patients with Graves' hyperthyroidism contributing to allergic bronchial asthma. Graves' disease can be associated with pulmonary arterial hypertension [24]. Studies have shown an association between Graves' disease treated with propylthiouracil and Wegener's granulomatosis [25]. Thyroid tuberculosis is a rare presentation of hyperthyroidism [26].

8. Skin

Common cutaneous manifestations of hyperthyroidism include flushing of the face, erythema of the palms, and hyperhidrosis of the palms and soles [27]. The epidermis becomes thin but not atrophic. Skin is warm, moist, and smooth. There is diffuse scalp hair thinning, and it has a downy texture.

Nails are soft, shiny, and onycholysis, or separation of the distal nail plate from the nail bed. The proximal portion of the nail plate is pink in color, and the distal portion changes to a white, opaque color. The nail plate is upturned, referred to as a Plummer's nail, and is most likely to be first seen on the fourth fingernail [28]. Thyroid acropachy, a rare manifestation of Graves' disease (0.1–1%), is characterized by the triad of digital clubbing, acral swelling, and diaphyseal proliferation of the periosteum in acral and distal long bones [29].

Pretibial myxedema is most commonly seen on the anterior tibia and dorsum of the feet. It includes sharply demarcated pink or purple-brown papules or nodules overlying a non-pitting thickening and induration. Other cutaneous manifestations of hyperthyroidism include chronic urticaria, dermographism, generalized pruritus, and eczematous dermatitis, which are less common [27].

9. Eyes

Stare and lid lag is common in hyperthyroidism. They are due to sympathetic overactivity, possibly mediated by increased alpha-adrenergic receptors in some tissues [30]. In lid lag, the sclera can be seen above the iris when the patient looks downward.

Patients with Graves' disease have orbitopathy characterized by inflammation of the extraocular muscles, orbital fat, and connective tissue. It can cause proptosis (exophthalmos), impairment of extraocular muscle function, and periorbital and conjunctival edema. Risk factors for Graves' orbitopathy are cigarette smoking, advancing age, and male sex [31].

10. Hematologic

In hyperthyroidism, red blood cell mass is increased. The plasma volume is also increased, resulting in a normochromic, normocytic anemia [32]. Autoimmune hematologic disorders such as immune thrombocytopenia (ITP) and pernicious anemia can be associated with Graves' disease. According to a meta-analysis, 10 percent of patients with Graves' hyperthyroidism can have neutropenia [33].

Hyperthyroidism can be a prothrombotic state [34]. Excess thyroid hormone was associated with a rise in prothrombotic factors, including factors VIII, IX, fibrinogen, von Willebrand factor, and plasminogen activator inhibitor-1 [35].

11. Genito-Urinary System

Urinary frequency and nocturia are common in hyperthyroidism. Possible causes include primary polydipsia [36] and hypercalciuria. Enuresis is common in children.

In women, high serum sex hormone-binding globulin (SHBG) concentrations result in high serum estradiol concentrations, low-normal serum free estradiol concentrations, and high serum luteinizing hormone (LH) concentrations, a reduced mid-cycle surge in LH secretion, oligomenorrhea, and anovulatory infertility [37, 38]. Amenorrhea can occur in women with severe hyperthyroidism.

In men, the increase in serum SHBG concentrations results in high serum total testosterone concentrations, but serum free (unbound) testosterone concentrations are normal or low [39, 40]. Serum LH concentrations may be slightly elevated. Extragonadal conversion of testosterone to estradiol is increased. These changes can cause gynecomastia, reduced libido, and erectile dysfunction [37, 41]. Spermatogenesis is often decreased or abnormal [40].

12. Metabolism and Endocrine System

Lipids: Patients with hyperthyroidism have low serum total and high-density lipoprotein (HDL) cholesterol concentrations and a low total cholesterol/HDL cholesterol ratio. These values usually increase after treatment [42].

Glucose: Hyperthyroidism interferes with glucose metabolism. It is associated with increased sensitivity of pancreatic beta cells to glucose, resulting in increased insulin secretion and antagonism to the peripheral action of insulin [43]. The latter effect usually predominates, leading to impaired glucose tolerance in untreated patients [44].

Adrenal: The hepatic inactivation of cortisol is accelerated. Serum cortisol-binding globulin (CBG) levels decrease, resulting in lower total serum cortisol concentrations. The urinary excretion of free cortisol can be normal or slightly increased.

Bone: Thyroid hormone stimulates bone resorption, resulting in increased porosity of cortical bone and reduced volume of trabecular bone [45]. Cortical bone density is lost greater than that of trabecular bone. As there is increased bone turnover, serum alkaline phosphatase and osteocalcin concentrations are high.

The increase in bone resorption leads to an increase in serum calcium concentrations, thereby inhibiting parathyroid hormone secretion and the conversion of calcidiol to calcitriol. There is an increased metabolic clearance rate of calcitriol. These changes lead to impaired calcium absorption and increased calcium excretion in urine. The net effect is osteoporosis and increased fracture risk in patients with chronic hyperthyroidism [46].

13. Thymus

In patients with Graves' disease, thymic enlargement due to hyperplasia has been reported [47, 48, 49]. Mechanisms postulated include autoimmune-mediated (thyroid-stimulating immunoglobulins from patients with Graves' disease bind to the thyroid-stimulating hormone [TSH] receptor in the human thymus and cause thymocyte proliferation) and hyperthyroidism-mediated (hyperthyroidism-induced angiogenesis) [47, 50].

Conclusion

Most common symptoms of hyperthyroidism include weight loss, tremors, anxiety, palpitations, intolerance to heat, diarrhea, etc. Patients with mild hyperthyroidism often have symptoms of one or only a few organ systems. Symptoms and signs of hyperthyroidism are more commonly seen in young patients than in the elderly. Older patients usually present with congestive heart failure, arrhythmias, and unexplained weight loss.

References

[1] Klein I, Ojamaa K. Thyroid hormone and the cardiovascular system. *N Engl J Med.* 2001;344(7):501-509.

[2] Marcisz C, Jonderko G, Wróblewski T, Kurzawska G, Mazur F. Left ventricular mass in patients with hyperthyroidism. *Med Sci Monit.* 2006 Nov;12(11):CR481-6. PMID: 17072274.

[3] Franklyn JA, Boelaert K. Thyrotoxicosis. *Lancet.* 2012; 379:1155-1166.

[4] Grais IM, Sowers JR. Thyroid and the heart. *Am J Med.* 2014;127(8):691-698.

[5] Danzi S, Klein I. Thyroid hormone and the cardiovascular system. *Med Clin North Am.* 2012 Mar;96(2):257-68. doi: 10.1016/j.mcna.2012.01.006. Epub 2012 Feb 14. PMID: 22443974.

[6] Iglesias P, Bajo MA, Selgas R, Díez JJ. Thyroid dysfunction and kidney disease: An update. *Rev Endocr Metab Disord.* 2017 Mar;18(1):131-144. doi: 10.1007/s11154-016-9395-7. PMID: 27864708.

[7] Kimmel M, Braun N, Alscher MD. Influence of thyroid function on different kidney function tests. *Kidney Blood Press Res.*2012; 1:9–17.

[8] Wang W, Li C, Summer SN, Falk S, Schrier RW. Polyuria of thyrotoxicosis: downregulation of aquaporin water channels and increased solute excretion. *Kidney Int.* 2007; 9:1088–94.

[9] Basu G, Mohapatra A. Interactions between thyroid disorders and kidney disease. *Indian J Endocrinol Metab*. 2012; 2:204–13.

[10] den Hollander JG, Wulkan RW, Mantel MJ, Berghout A. Correlation between severity of thyroid dysfunction and renal function. *Clin Endocrinol*. 2005; 4: 423–7.

[11] Feldman AZ, Shrestha RT, Hennessey JV. Neuropsychiatric manifestations of thyroid disease. *Endocrinol Metab Clin North Am*. 2013;42(3):453-476.

[12] Rieben C, Segna D, da Costa BR, Collet TH, Chaker L, Aubert CE, Baumgartner C, Almeida OP, Hogervorst E, Trompet S, Masaki K, Mooijaart SP, Gussekloo J, Peeters RP, Bauer DC, Aujesky D, Rodondi N. Subclinical Thyroid Dysfunction and the Risk of Cognitive Decline: a Meta-Analysis of Prospective Cohort Studies. *J Clin Endocrinol Metab*. 2016 Dec;101(12):4945-4954. doi: 10.1210/jc.2016-2129. Epub 2016 Sep 30. PMID: 27689250; PMCID: PMC6287525.

[13] Ladd JM, Sabsabi B, von Oettingen JE. Thyroid Storm in a Toddler Presenting as a Febrile Seizure. *Pediatrics*. 2020 Feb;145(2):e20191920. doi: 10.1542/peds. 2019-1920. PMID: 31980544.

[14] Thamprajamchit S, Jariengprasert C, Rajatanavin R. Propylthiouracil-induced sensorineural hearing loss associated with antineutrophil cytoplasmic antibodies. *Endocr Pract* 2004;10(5):432–437.

[15] Sahni V, Gupta N, Anuradha S, Tatke M, Kar P. Thyrotoxic neuropathy- an under diagnosed condition. *Med J Malaysia*. 2007 Mar;62(1):76-7. PMID: 17682580.

[16] Masannat Y, Gandhy R, Olajide O, Kheetan R, Yaqub A. Chorea associated with thyrotoxicosis due to toxic multinodular goiter. *Thyroid*. 2011 Nov;21(11):1279-80. doi: 10.1089/thy.2011.0018. Epub 2011 Sep 21. PMID: 21936672.

[17] Bartley GB, Fatourechi V, Kadrmas EF, Jacobsen SJ, Ilstrup DM, Garrity JA, Gorman CA. Clinical features of Graves' ophthalmopathy in an incidence cohort. *Am J Ophthalmol*. 1996 Mar;121(3):284-90. doi: 10.1016/s0002-9394(14)70276-4. PMID: 8597271.

[18] Puri V, Chaudhry N. Paroxysmal kinesigenic dyskinesia manifestation of hyperthyroidism. *Neurol India*. 2004 Mar;52(1):102-3. PMID: 15069252.

[19] Ebert, Ellen C. MD The Thyroid and the Gut, *Journal of Clinical Gastroenterology:* July 2010 - Volume 44 - Issue 6 - p 402-406 doi: 10.1097/ MCG.0b013e3181d6bc3e.

[20] Boelaert K, Newby PR, Simmonds MJ, Holder RL, Carr-Smith JD, Heward JM, Manji N, Allahabadia A, Armitage M, Chatterjee KV, Lazarus JH, Pearce SH, Vaidya B, Gough SC, Franklyn JA. Prevalence and relative risk of other autoimmune diseases in subjects with autoimmune thyroid disease. *Am J Med*. 2010 Feb;123(2):183.e1-9. doi: 10.1016/j.amjmed.2009.06.030. PMID: 20103030.

[21] Tsatsoulis A, Johnson EO, Kalogera CH, Seferiadis K, Tsolas O. The effect of thyrotoxicosis on adrenocortical reserve. *Eur J Endocrinol*. 2000 Mar;142(3):231-5. doi: 10.1530/eje.0.1420231. PMID: 10700716.

[22] Oki K, Yamane K, Koide J, Mandai K, Nakanishi S, Fujikawa R, Kohno N. A case of polyglandular autoimmune syndrome type III complicated with autoimmune hepatitis. *Endocr J*. 2006 Oct;53(5):705-9. doi: 10.1507/endocrj.k05-166. Epub 2006 Sep 1. PMID: 16946565.

[23] Goswami R, Guleria R, Gupta AK, Gupta N, Marwaha RK, Pande JN, Kochupillai N. Prevalence of diaphragmatic muscle weakness and dyspnoea in Graves' disease and their reversibility with carbimazole therapy. *Eur J Endocrinol.* 2002 Sep;147(3):299-303. doi: 10.1530/eje.0.1470299. PMID: 12213666.

[24] Ismail HM. Reversible pulmonary hypertension and isolated right-sided heart failure associated with hyperthyroidism. *J Gen Intern Med.* 2007;22(1):148-150.

[25] Zimmerman L. Pulmonary complications of endocrine diseases. In: Broaddus VC, Mason RJ, Ernst JD, King TE, Lazarus SC, Murray JF, Nadel JA, Slutsky AS, Gotway MB (eds). *Murray and Nadel's. Textbook of respiratory medicine.* 6th Edition, Philadelphia: Elsevier Saunders, 2016; chapter 95: 1671-1678.

[26] Bansal LK, Gupta S, Gupta AK, Chaudhary P. Thyroid tuberculosis. *Indian J Tuberc.* 2021 Apr;68(2):272-278. doi: 10.1016/j.ijtb.2020.09.006. Epub 2020 Sep 12. PMID: 33845964.

[27] Jabbour SA. Cutaneous manifestations of endocrine disorders: a guide for dermatologists. *Am J Clin Dermatol* 2003; 4:315-31.

[28] Rustin MH. Andrews' diseases of the skin – clinical dermatology. *Postgrad Med J* 1990;66:984.

[29] Lause M, Kamboj A, Fernandez Faith E. Dermatologic manifestations of endocrine disorders. *Transl Pediatr.* 2017;6(4):300-312. doi:10.21037/tp.2017. 09.08.

[30] Bilezikian JP, Loeb JN. The influence of hyperthyroidism and hypothyroidism on alpha- and beta-adrenergic receptor systems and adrenergic responsiveness. *Endocr Rev.* 1983 Fall;4(4):378-88. doi: 10.1210/edrv-4-4-378. PMID: 6317368.

[31] Lee MH, Chin YH, Ng CH, Nistala KRY, Ow ZGW, Sundar G, Yang SP, Khoo CM. Risk Factors of Thyroid Eye Disease. *Endocr Pract.* 2021 Mar;27(3):245-253. doi: 10.1016/j.eprac.2020.11.011. Epub 2020 Dec 14. PMID: 33655885.

[32] Nightingale S, Vitek PJ, Himsworth RL. The haematology of hyperthyroidism. *Q J Med.* 1978 Jan;47(185):35-47. PMID: 674549.

[33] Scappaticcio L, Maiorino MI, Maio A, Esposito K, Bellastella G. Neutropenia in patients with hyperthyroidism: Systematic review and meta-analysis. *Clin Endocrinol* (Oxf). 2021 Mar;94(3):473-483. doi: 10.1111/cen.14313. Epub 2020 Sep 1. PMID: 32799342.

[34] Franchini M, Lippi G, Targher G. Hyperthyroidism and venous thrombosis: a casual or causal association? A systematic literature review. *Clin Appl Thromb Hemost.* 2011 Aug;17(4):387-92. doi: 10.1177/1076029610364521. Epub 2010 Mar 22. PMID: 20308227.

[35] Stuijver DJ, van Zaane B, Romualdi E, Brandjes DP, Gerdes VE, Squizzato A. The effect of hyperthyroidism on procoagulant, anticoagulant and fibrinolytic factors: a systematic review and meta-analysis. *Thromb Haemost.* 2012 Dec;108(6):1077-88. doi: 10.1160/TH12-07-0496. Epub 2012 Sep 26. PMID: 23014708.

[36] Evered DC, Hayter CJ, Surveyor I. Primary polydipsia in thyrotoxicosis. *Metabolism.* 1972 May;21(5):393-404. doi: 10.1016/0026-0495(72)90052-2. PMID: 4111512.

[37] Ridgway EC, Maloof F, Longcope C. Androgen and oestrogen dynamics in hyperthyroidism. *J Endocrinol.* 1982 Oct;95(1):105-15. doi: 10.1677/joe.0. 0950105. PMID: 7130886.

[38] Koutras DA. Disturbances of menstruation in thyroid disease. *Ann N Y Acad Sci.* 1997 Jun 17;816:280-4. doi: 10.1111/j.1749-6632.1997.tb52152.x. PMID: 9238278.

[39] Hudson RW, Edwards AL. Testicular function in hyperthyroidism. *J Androl.* 1992 Mar-Apr;13(2):117-24. PMID: 1597395.

[40] Abalovich M, Levalle O, Hermes R, Scaglia H, Aranda C, Zylbersztein C, Oneto A, Aquilano D, Gutierrez S. Hypothalamic-pituitary-testicular axis and seminal parameters in hyperthyroid males. *Thyroid.* 1999 Sep;9(9):857-63. doi: 10.1089/thy.1999.9.857. PMID: 10524563.

[41] Carani C, Isidori AM, Granata A, Carosa E, Maggi M, Lenzi A, Jannini EA. Multicenter study on the prevalence of sexual symptoms in male hypo- and hyperthyroid patients. *J Clin Endocrinol Metab.* 2005 Dec;90(12):6472-9. doi: 10.1210/jc.2005-1135. Epub 2005 Oct 4. PMID: 16204360.

[42] O'Brien T, Katz K, Hodge D, Nguyen TT, Kottke BA, Hay ID. The effect of the treatment of hypothyroidism and hyperthyroidism on plasma lipids and apolipoproteins AI, AII and E. *Clin Endocrinol* (Oxf). 1997 Jan;46(1):17-20. doi: 10.1046/j.1365-2265.1997.d01-1753.x. PMID: 9059553.

[43] Reasner CA. Autoimmune thyroid disease and type 1 diabetes. *Diabetes Reviews.* 1993; 1:343.

[44] Andersen OO, Friis T, Ottesen B. Glucose tolerance and insulin secretion in hyperthyroidism. *Acta Endocrinol* (Copenh). 1977 Mar;84(3):576-87. doi: 10.1530/acta.0.0840576. PMID: 320805.

[45] Ross DS. Hyperthyroidism, thyroid hormone therapy, and bone. *Thyroid.* 1994 Fall;4(3):319-26. doi: 10.1089/thy.1994.4.319. PMID: 7833670.

[46] Williams GR, Bassett JHD. Thyroid diseases and bone health. *J Endocrinol Invest.* 2018 Jan;41(1):99-109. doi: 10.1007/s40618-017-0753-4. Epub 2017 Aug 29. PMID: 28853052; PMCID: PMC5754375.

[47] Dalla Costa M, Mangano FA, Betterle C. Thymic hyperplasia in patients with Graves' disease. *J Endocrinol Invest.* 2014 Dec;37(12):1175-9. doi: 10.1007/s40618-014-0157-7. Epub 2014 Aug 23. PMID: 25149085.

[48] Yacoub A, Gaitonde DY, Wood JC. Thymic hyperplasia and Graves disease: management of anterior mediastinal masses in patients with Graves disease. *Endocr Pract.* 2009 Sep-Oct;15(6):534-9. doi: 10.4158/EP09025.ORR. PMID: 19491074.

[49] Huang W, Molitch ME. Enlarged thymus in a patient with dyspnea and weight loss. *JAMA.* 2015 Jun 2;313(21):2174-5. doi: 10.1001/jama.2015.2713. PMID: 26034958.

[50] Wortsman J, McConnachie P, Baker JR Jr, Burman KD. Immunoglobulins that cause thymocyte proliferation from a patient with Graves' disease and an enlarged thymus. *Am J Med.* 1988 Jul;85(1):117-21. doi: 10.1016/0002-9343(88)90516-5. PMID: 3260449.

Chapter 5

The Evaluation of Patients with Hyperthyroidism

K. V. S. Hari Kumar[1,*], MD, DNB
Consultant Endocrinologist, MAGNA Clinic, Hyderabad, India

Abstract

Thyrotoxicosis with diffuse thyroid disease is caused by either Graves' disease or destructive thyrotoxicosis. The evaluation of patients includes detailed history, detailed clinical examination with special emphasis on the goiter, eyes, skin and nails. Clinical features of hyperthyroidism include almost all the major and minor organs of the body. The pattern of involvement and the severity help us in the differential diagnosis of thyrotoxicosis. The diagnosis of florid Graves' disease is easy in the clinic, whereas, it is difficult to distinguish between the early Graves' disease and destructive thyroiditis clinically. This differentiation is essential as the antithyroid drugs are indicated in the former and not in the later condition. The diagnostic modalities that help in the differential diagnosis of hyperthyroidism include thyroid function tests, thyroid autoantibodies, color flow doppler imaging of the thyroid and pertechnetate uptake thyroid scan. In this chapter, I shall present the clinical and laboratory evaluation of the patients with hyperthyroidism along with the suggested diagnostic algorithm.

Keywords: hyperthyroidism, thyrotoxicosis, thyroid storm, destructive thyroiditis

---

* Corresponding Author's Email: hariendo@gmail.com.

In: Understanding and Managing Hyperthyroidism
Editor: Poongkodi Karunakaran
ISBN: 979-8-88697-636-6

Introduction

Thyrotoxicosis is defined as a clinical condition due to excess thyroid hormones in the circulation, and hyperthyroidism denotes that the origin of these excess hormones is from a hyperactive thyroid gland. Determining the etiologies of hyperthyroidism is essential to plan a proper and definite therapy. Graves' disease (GD), Toxic multinodular goiter (TMNG), Solitary Toxic Adenoma (STA), and Destructive Thyroiditis (DT) are the commonest causes of thyrotoxicosis in clinical practice [1]. Screening the general population for thyrotoxicosis is not recommended by any guidelines, and the testing should be done in patients with suggestive clinical symptoms only.

1. Clinical Assessment

The diagnosis of hyperthyroidism is generally straightforward in a typical patient with classical symptoms and signs of thyrotoxicosis. However, in view of the minimal correlation between the structural and functional alterations in the thyroid hormones, the clinical diagnosis is often difficult and diagnostic aids are often indispensable [2]. The standard classification of various conditions leading to thyrotoxicosis with or without hyperthyroidism is shown in Figure 1. The differentiation is important as each of these conditions is managed differently, and beyond the therapy, the underlying etiology also helps in the long-term prognostication of the patient. The accurate diagnosis also helps select the appropriate treatment for female patients who have to plan their pregnancy.

Clinical assessment is often misleading or less contributory in the presence of thyrotoxicosis during pregnancy and in elderly patients. During the first trimester of pregnancy, the elevated levels of human chorionic gonadotropin stimulate the thyroid gland leading to a condition known as "Gestational Thyrotoxicosis". This is a self-limiting condition and it is essential to differentiate this from GD as the antithyroid drugs are indicated in the latter and not in the former [3]. Elderly patients may not have the classical features of thyrotoxicosis and present with fatigue, listlessness, atrial fibrillation, weight loss, and depression. This condition is known as "Apathetic thyrotoxicosis" and often requires detailed biochemical and nuclear imaging tests for the diagnosis [4]. Hence, it is essential to look at the clinical setting closely and take the help of diagnostic aids in the evaluation of patients with hyperthyroidism.

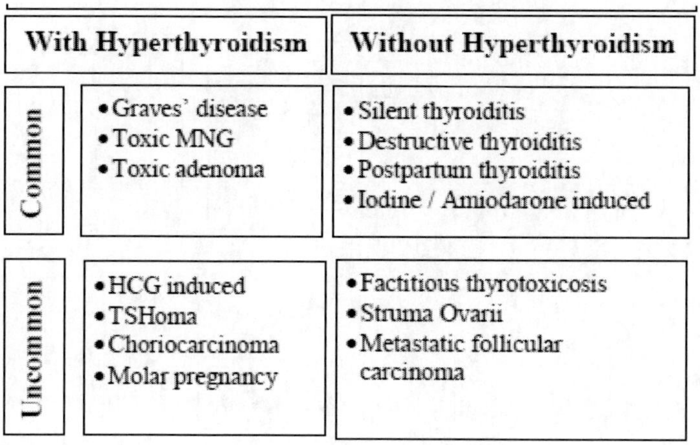

Figure 1. Etiologies of thyrotoxicosis.

1.1. Clinical Clues

The clinical approach toward a patient with hyperthyroidism is to identify the underlying etiology and assess the severity in order to suggest appropriate therapy. Many patients may have classical diagnostic clinical features and do not require further testing to confirm the diagnosis. In a patient presenting with palpitations, weight loss, hyper defecation over a few months, and examination revealing the presence of tachycardia, goiter, and ophthalmopathy, the diagnosis of GD is evident, and further testing is not warranted. However, such classical presentation is not often observed in practice. The typical clinical profile and setting that suggests underlying diagnosis along with relevant diagnostic aids is given in Table 1.

TMNG is more common in iodine-deficient areas and typically occurs in middle-aged individuals with a long-standing history of goiter. The features of thyrotoxicosis in TMNG are more subtle, unlike that of the GD. STAs are present in young individuals from iodine-deficient areas, and symptoms may be variable in presentation. DT produces an abrupt onset of thyrotoxic symptoms, especially after a brief viral illness, and symptoms may resolve within a few weeks. The symptoms are maximum in the initial week of the illness, and many patients may complain of throat pain and have tenderness. The initial thyrotoxic phase of autoimmune thyroiditis is known as the "Hashitoxicosis" [5]. This condition also has maximum clinical features initially and modifies towards hypothyroidism in a few weeks.

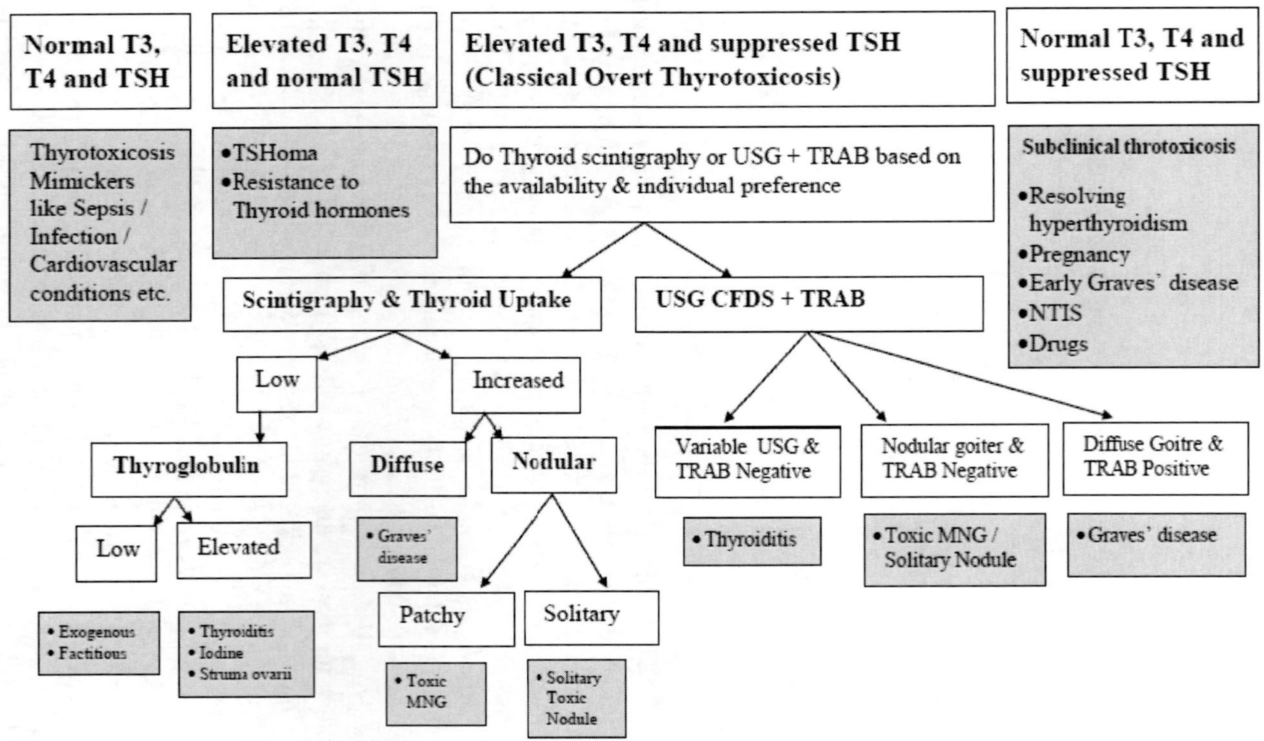

Figure 2. Clinical features of suspected thyrotoxicosis & T3, T4 and TSH.

Table 1. Salient features of Thyrotoxicosis

Clinical features	Biochemical observations	Other diagnostic findings
• Goiter, Ophthalmopathy • Thyroid acropachy • Pretibial Myxedema	• Elevated T3/T4 ratio > 20 • Transaminitis • TRAB Positive	• Increased RAIU • Increased Vascularity
• Immediately after delivery • Mild goiter • No eye signs	• T3/T4 ratio < 20 • TPO antibody may be positive • TRAB negative	• Low uptake • Heterogenous echotexture with reduced gland vascularity
• Throat pain, Malaise, Fever • Thyroid tenderness	• T3/T4 ratio < 20 • TPO Positive	• Low uptake • Reduced vascularity
• H/O offending drug intake	• T3/T4 ratio < 20 • TPO negative	• Low uptake scan • USG not required
• Palpable thyroid with multiple nodules, Non tender • Asymmetric goiter	• T3/T4 ratio > 20 • TPO may be Positive	• Patchy increased Uptake • Heterogeneously increased vascularity
• Goiter • CNS symptoms • Mild features of thyrotoxicosis	• Unsuppressed TSH with elevated T3 and T4 • Other anterior pituitary hormone involvement	• Mild increased uptake • Sellar mass
• Goiter, Deafness • Positive family history	• Unsuppressed TSH with elevated T3 and T4	• No characteristic findings on imaging

1.2. Disease Severity

Clinical assessment is the only modality to assess the severity of thyrotoxicosis. None of the biochemical tests or imaging findings help classify the thyrotoxicosis severity. The presence of cardiovascular and neuromuscular symptoms suggests a diagnosis of severe thyrotoxicosis, and the management has to be planned accordingly. The severity of thyrotoxicosis is assessed by a clinical score known as Burch – Wartofsky score [6]. It consists of five parameters (fever, cardiovascular, neurological, and gastrointestinal features along with the history of precipitating event) which are scored as per the clinical finding as shown in Table 2. A total score of less than 25 rules out the thyroid storm, whereas a score above 45 is highly suggestive of a thyroid storm. Patients with a score between 25 and 44 support the thyroid storm diagnosis.

Table 2. Bursch – Wartofsky Clinical scoring system

System	Features	Points
Temperature	99 – 104^{0}F	5 – 30
CNS disturbance	Agitation, delirium, Coma	0 – 30
GI disturbance	Diarrhoea, Pain, Vomiting, Jaundice	0 – 15
CVS dysfunction	Tachycardia, Atrial fibrillation, Failure	5 – 35
Precipitating event	Present/Absent	0 – 10

2. Biochemical Evaluation

The diagnostic workup of any patient with hyperthyroidism begins with estimating the thyroid hormones. The commonly estimated thyroid panel includes thyroid stimulating hormone (TSH), thyroxine (T4), and triiodothyronine (T3). Thyroid hormones are bound to albumin, transthyretin, and thyroid-binding globulin in the serum. T4 and T3 levels are also affected by the changes in the concentration of their binding proteins. Hence, in certain situations, free T3 and free T4 (unbound fractions) are used for the diagnosis. Other biochemical changes in thyrotoxicosis lend support to the diagnosis, and thyroid antibodies also aid in the diagnosis.

2.1. Thyroid Hormones

TSH is the best initial test for thyrotoxicosis as the assays for the same are standardized, accurate, and available across the country. Moreover, TSH has the highest sensitivity and specificity as a single test to diagnose thyrotoxicosis [7]. This is because of the log-linear relation between the thyroid hormones and TSH, which implies that even a minor change in the thyroid hormones is reflected in the TSH. The diagnosis of thyrotoxicosis is confirmed with the detection of elevated thyroid hormones and suppressed TSH. Elevated thyroid hormones with suppressed TSH are known as overt thyrotoxicosis, whereas normal thyroid hormones with suppressed TSH are known as subclinical thyrotoxicosis. The approach to patients with subclinical thyrotoxicosis is similar to that of overt thyrotoxicosis.

T3 is the active thyroid hormone, and T4 is the prehormone, which is converted into T3 in the target tissues. A normally functioning thyroid gland produces 90% of T4 and 10% of T3, which may vary during intense stimulation of the thyroid gland. The ratio of T4 to T3 is also proposed as a differentiating feature of thyrotoxicosis. A hyperactive gland produces more T3, whereas more preformed T4 is released in cases of DT. Hence, the T3/T4 ratio (ng/μg) of more than 20 is suggestive of GD, and a ratio of less than 20 is suggestive of DT [8]. Patients with iatrogenic/factitious thyrotoxicosis have a high ratio of T4/T3 due to the ingestion of T4. About 1% of patients with hyperthyroidism may present with elevated T3, normal T4, and suppressed TSH. This condition is known as T3 toxicosis and may be due to an early stage of GD or STA [9].

Another important feature during the evaluation of thyroid hormones is the presence of elevated thyroid hormones with normal TSH. This clinical condition is known as "Euthyroid Hyperthyroxinemia" and has a variety of causes, predominantly due to the changes in the thyroid binding proteins [10]. This is seen in patients with elevated T4 binding globulin (TBG) or transthyretin and in the presence of abnormal forms of albumin, which binds strongly with the T4 (known as familial dysalbuminemic hyperthyroxinemia). TBG is elevated in hyperestrogenic states like pregnancy and consumption of estrogen containing pills, hepatitis, or inherited as an X-linked trait. Other conditions that may lead to euthyroid hyperthyroxinemia include acute psychosis, extremely high altitude, drugs like propranolol, amiodarone, and amphetamine abuse. In such situations, it is always better to look at the free thyroid hormones to identify thyrotoxicosis. However, it should always be borne in mind that the assay for the free thyroid hormones is less validated than the estimation of the total thyroid hormones. Spurious elevation of free thyroid hormones is observed in the presence of heterophilic antibodies that interfere with the assay and also in the setting of the heparin therapy.

Unsuppressed TSH with elevated thyroid hormones is a rarity and denotes the presence of either pituitary TSH secreting tumor (TSHoma) or resistance to thyroid hormone (RTH) [11]. The detailed clinical profile would give the clues for these conditions, and the other associated hormonal changes aid in clinching the diagnosis. TSHoma may have mild thyrotoxicosis features and other central features like headache, vomiting, and involvement of other hormonal axes. RTH is a syndrome of reduced end-organ responsiveness to the thyroid hormones and may involve other family members. Antithyroid drugs worsen the condition further, and clinicians must be aware of these conditions, especially in the setting of clinical and biochemical discordance.

2.2. Thyroid Antibodies

The thyroid antibodies available for estimation in clinical practice include thyroid peroxidase (TPO), thyroglobulin (TG), and TSH receptor antibody (TRAB). Out of the above mentioned three antibodies, the detection of TRAB has the highest sensitivity and specificity for the diagnosis of GD [12]. TPO antibodies are present in two-third of patients with GD and lymphocytic thyroiditis and are not necessary for the diagnosis. The positive TPO suggests the underlying autoimmune status but does not confirm the diagnosis of GD, unlike the TRAB. TG antibodies are routinely not used in the evaluation of thyrotoxicosis. They are helpful in patients with functional metastatic thyroid cancer after surgery and radio ablation to check for the thyroglobulin level estimation.

TRAB is estimated using either an immunological assay or biological assays. The biological assays are the definite way of diagnosing the condition as the TRAB can have stimulating, blocking, or neutral effects on the TSH receptor. The type of the antibody (stimulating or blocking) is determined by the production of the cyclic AMP in the biological assays using cultured cells. The antibodies may have varying activity between stimulating and blocking type during the natural course of the disease. Antibody assays assess the presence of immunoglobulins that can block the binding of the TSH receptor in an in-vitro preparation. Few patients may have TSH stimulating and blocking antibodies concurrently and have a mild disease spectrum of GD. The limitation of using immunological assays is they do not reveal the underlying biological activity of the antibody.

Management guidelines by the major societies recommend the use of the TRABs as the 1st step in the approach to a patient with thyrotoxicosis [13]. However, the same test is not widely available and is expensive. The 1st and 2nd-generation TRAB assays have low sensitivity and specificity. The 3rd generation assays use a human monoclonal TSH receptor stimulating antibody and have a high sensitivity and specificity in the diagnosis of GD. TRAB is rarely positive in a few cases of subacute thyroiditis but is pathognomonic of GD. The TRAB are strongly positive in GD and weakly positive in other conditions, and the titer of the positivity could also be used in the differential diagnosis. TRAB estimation also helps predict relapse in patients after discontinuation of antithyroid drugs and the risk of neonatal thyrotoxicosis as they readily cross the placenta.

2.3. Ancillary Tests

The circulating excess of thyroid hormones affects other biochemical parameters, especially in patients with the long-standing disease. Other biochemical features in patients with hyperthyroidism include normocytic normochromic anemia, lymphocytosis, hypercalcemia, transaminitis, and elevated alkaline phosphatase. The baseline estimation of liver function is essential to rule out an idiosyncratic reaction of acute hepatitis after starting the antithyroid drugs. Hyperthyroidism affects the bone significantly, and many patients have evidence of bone loss and an increase in the bone turnover markers [14]. In elderly patients with thyrotoxicosis, it is essential to evaluate the bone mineral density. In case of significant bone loss, bisphosphonates may be considered along with the management of hyperthyroidism.

A detailed cardiac evaluation, including electrocardiogram, echocardiography, and Holter monitoring, may be necessary for elderly patients with thyrotoxicosis. This is because of the need to use beta-blockers in high doses for patients with GD, which may have an effect on the underlying cardiac function. Elderly patients with thyrotoxicosis are prone to rhythm abnormalities, including atrial fibrillation, and some of them may require the use of anticoagulant therapy additionally. Hence, a detailed systemic evaluation of all the biochemical tests is necessary for most of the patients with thyrotoxicosis.

3. Etiological Diagnosis

In patients with no diagnostic features clinically, nuclear imaging helps in the etiological diagnosis. In situations where the nuclear imaging is contraindicated, ultrasonography is of help, and histopathology is never used for diagnosing the etiology of thyrotoxicosis.

3.1. Nuclear Imaging

Radioactive iodine uptake (RAIU) is the imaging modality of choice for the evaluation of thyrotoxicosis [15]. The technique involves administering a small dose of radioiodine and estimating the percentage uptake by the thyroid gland at a fixed interval of usually 24 hr. In recent times, nuclear imaging is done using Technetium, as the imaging can be obtained within 20 minutes after the injection. However, clinicians ordering this test should understand that technetium is only trapped by the thyroid gland and not organified. Based on the scan findings, patients with thyrotoxicosis may be classified as diffusely increased uptake suggestive of GD, patchy increased uptake suggestive of TMNG, and a solitary area of increased uptake with suppression of the tracer in the surrounding areas leading to the diagnosis of STA.

The major advantage of thyroid scintigraphy is to delineate the thyrotoxic patients with hyperthyroidism (increased uptake) and without hyperthyroidism (low uptake), as shown in table 1. In a thyrotoxic patient without orbitopathy, it is mandatory to identify the underlying etiology using either TRAB or nuclear imaging. The RAIU may be spuriously low in patients with recent exposure to either iodine and iodine-containing compounds like contrast media or seaweed soup etc. In a patient with suspected iodine exposure affecting the results of the RAIU, it is advised to check for the urine iodine concentration. In patients with struma ovarii (hyperfunctioning thyroid tissue in the ovarian teratoma), the uptake may be absent in the neck region and increased in the pelvis. The co-existence of GD and TMNG may occasionally be seen in a few patients known as the Marine-Lenhart syndrome. The scan may show a heterogenous intake with a background of increased uptake, and these patients are ideally treated with radioiodine therapy if not contraindicated.

3.2. Ultrasonography

Ultrasonography (USG) of the thyroid gland also helps in the differential diagnosis of thyrotoxicosis. The ease of testing, wide availability, and the immediate results help this diagnostic modality as the initial investigation of thyrotoxicosis in the developing world [16]. Moreover, USG is beneficial in certain situations where the RAIU scan is contraindicated like pregnancy and lactation [17]. Gray scale USG may not help in the differentiation and this require the use of the colour flow doppler sonography (CFDS). The hypervascular thyroid gland and increased blood flow of the thyroid arteries help in identifying the patients with GD. In patients with DT, the blood flow is not increased and the peak systolic velocity (PSV) of the inferior thyroid artery is below 40 cm/sec. USG and CFDS also helps in the differentiation of the subtypes of the amiodarone induced thyrotoxicosis also in which the PSV is increased in Type 1 and reduced in type 2. Technical expertise and checking for the artefacts are few limitations of the USG for the assessment of thyrotoxicosis. The results have to be interpreted with the underlying iodine adequacy status. In patients with severe iodine deficiency the gland is hypervascular and may mimic the sonological features of the GD. In addition to the diagnosis, the USG helps in the serial follow up of these patients as the vascularity changes parallel that of the biochemical changes of the thyroid gland.

USG also helps in identifying the nodular disease, presence of MNG, diffuse involvement of thyroid parenchyma or any other feature atypical of thyrotoxicosis. The USG is more helpful in documenting the suspicious nodule for a FNAC. As a general rule, any over functioning thyroid nodule (also known as STA) has minimal chances of being malignant in nature. However, the functioning of the nodule is more evident by the radionuclide imaging.

3.3. Histopathology

During the evaluation of thyrotoxicosis, histopathological examination of the thyroid tissue is not required. However, in patients with suspicious malignancy in a nodular disease in the background of thyrotoxicosis, the FNAC (Fine needle aspiration cytology) is the most accurate way of identifying thyroid malignancy. Functioning thyroid nodules with thyrotoxicosis are not subjected for the FNAC as the incidence of malignancy is low in these patients. USG doesn't differentiate between the benign and malignant nodules and it is better to perform the FNAC. The treatment approach is based on the individual characteristics and surgical options may be considered over the medical management.

The thyroid specimens have been studied in patients with thyrotoxicosis, where the gland is removed as part of therapy or in suspected malignancy. In GD, the follicles are hyperplastic with prominent papillary infoldings along with columnar lining epithelium [18]. TMNG has a typical appearance with variable sized dilated follicles with flattened hyperplastic epithelium and also hemosiderin deposition suggesting evidence of old haemorrhage in the nodule. There can be variable mixture of the granulomatous response, fibrosis and calcification in the nodules.

4. Diagnostic Approach

The diagnostic algorithm of hyperthyroidism involves a detailed history, biochemical confirmation using the thyroid hormone panel and further testing as per the requirement. The approach to a patient is given in the flow chart given as Figure 2. In a patient with elevated thyroid hormones, unsuppressed TSH effectively excludes the diagnosis of thyrotoxicosis with few exceptions like RTH or TSHoma leading to thyrotoxicosis. The approach is modified as per the clinical features, availability of the tests, socioeconomic situation and need of confirmation of the diagnosis. Many guidelines recommend doing thyroid scintigraphy if the 3rd generation TRAB tests are not available. American guidelines recommend using the thyroid scintigraphy as the initial test if the diagnosis of GD is not clinically established [13]. Scintigraphy is also recommended in patients with a nodular goitre in presence of hyperthyroidism and clinical profile suggestive of TMNG or STA. However, European and Asian guidelines suggest use of the USG along with TRAB for the diagnosis [19, 20]. The differences in the guidelines also stem from the fact that the predominant reason of the thyrotoxicosis is nodular goiter in Europe & Asians, whereas, the GD is predominant in the America.

The DD of thyrotoxicosis is complex in certain special situations. GD can develop in patients with a pre-existing nodular goiter and thyroid nodules may develop in patients with long standing GD. Patients with TMNG may have TRAB positivity and coexistence of the GD and TMG can be found in the same patient which is known as the Marine-Lenhart syndrome. These are the situations where the diagnostic tests are further confusing and the clinical judgement plays an important role in the selection of appropriate therapy. TRAB have a sensitivity of 96% and specificity of 99% for the diagnosis of GD. In patients with a nodular goitre and TRAB weakly positive, it is better to do a thyroid scintigraphy to arrive at the diagnosis. In order to diagnose the etiology of hyperthyroidism correctly, it is essential to know the iodine status of the population. It is important to understand the limitations and strengths of each modality and not rely on only one of the methods exclusively for the diagnosis. Table 3 enumerates the available diagnostic modalities and the clinical settings in which they are helpful in the evaluation. The essence of practice lies in the judicious use of the available resources and to establish the diagnosis.

Table 3. Diagnostic modalities and their indications during evaluation of thyrotoxicosis

S.No	Diagnostic Modality	Clinical Indications
1.	T3 T4 TSH	Initial screening test of thyrotoxicosis
2.	Thyroglobulin	Suspected Thyroiditis
3.	TRAB	Diagnosis of GD Prediction of Neonatal thyrotoxicosis Assessment of remission during GD management Euthyroid Graves Orbitopathy
4.	TPO Antibody	Confirmation of Hashitoxicosis and GD Predicts risk of SAT/Postpartum Thyroiditis
5.	RAIU/Technetium Pertechnate scan	Confirmation of Graves' disease (High uptake)
6.	USG/CFDS	Suspicion of GD/SAT/GTT Thyrotoxicosis during Pregnancy/Lactation
7.	Whole body Iodine Scan	Suspected Struma Ovarii/Functioning Metastatic thyroid follicular carcinoma
8.	HCG levels	Suspected Gestational Thyrotoxicosis, hyperemesis gravidarum, molar pregnancy, testicular tumour, choriocarcinoma

5. Diagnostic Pitfalls

Clinical features that mimic thyrotoxicosis are seen in patients with sepsis, infections, anxiety, chronic fatigue, and pheochromocytoma. The clinical setting is evident in all these conditions to arrive at the diagnosis and thyroid hormone panel is enough to distinguish from these conditions. Few conditions which may cause low TSH with variable T4 levels include NTIS, gestational toxicosis, central hypothyroidism and use of drugs like Dopamine, Glucocorticoids, bexarotene, mitotane etc.

Biotin is a common supplement in many multivitamin preparations and is used in high doses for managing the hair fall and brittle nails. Biotin is a key reagent in many of the assays and can interfere with the result of the thyroid hormone [20]. The use of high dose biotin produced a thyroid hormone profile similar to that of thyrotoxicosis. It is important to take a detailed drug history and patients are advised to stop all the supplements for at least 72 hours and repeat the test in case of mismatch between the clinical and biochemical picture.

Conclusion

To conclude, the evaluation of a patient with thyrotoxicosis is often simple and may not require laborious testing. In atypical patients, the evaluation is complex and requires elaborate testing to determine the underlying etiological diagnosis. Clinicians should discern the cause from clinical features along with the diagnostic aids like scintigraphy, USG and antibody testing as appropriate. The practitioners have to be aware of the diagnostic pitfalls to prevent misdiagnosis of thyrotoxicosis.

References

[1] De Leo S, Lee SY, Braverman LE. Hyperthyroidism. *Lancet.* 2016 27; 388(10047): 906-918.

[2] Smith TJ, Hegedu¨ s L. Graves' disease. *N Engl J Med.* 2016; 375:1552-65.

[3] Cooper DS, Laurberg P. Hyperthyroidism in pregnancy. *Lancet Diabetes Endocrinol* 2013; 1:238–249.

[4] Boelaert K, Torlinska B, Holder RL, Franklyn JA. Older subjects with hyperthyroidism present with a paucity of symptoms and signs: a large cross sectional study. *J Clin Endocrinol Metab* 2010; 95:2715-26.

[5] Shahbaz A, Aziz K, Umair M, Sachmechi I. Prolonged Duration of Hashitoxicosis in a Patient with Hashimoto's Thyroiditis: A Case Report and Review of Literature. *Cureus.* 2018;10(6):e2804.

[6] Burch HB, Wartofsky L. Life-threatening thyrotoxicosis. Thyroid storm. *Endocrinol Metab Clin North Am* 1993; 22:263–77.

[7] de los Santos ET, Starich GH, Mazzaferri EL. Sensitivity, specificity, and cost-effectiveness of the sensitive thyrotropin assay in the diagnosis of thyroid disease in ambulatory patients. *Arch Intern Med* 1989; 149:526–532.

[8] Carle A, Knudsen N, Pedersen IB, Perrild H, Ovesen L, Rasmussen LB, Laurberg P. Determinants of serum T4 and T3 at the time of diagnosis in nosological types of thyrotoxicosis: a population-based study. *Eur J Endocrinol* 2013; 169:537–545.

[9] Jaroudi S, Gavin M, Boylan K, Peiris AN. Transient T3 toxicosis associated with Hashimoto's disease. *Proc (Bayl Univ Med Cent).* 2018; 32(1):80-81.

[10] Borst GC, Eil C, Burman KD. Euthyroid hyperthyroxinemia. *Ann Intern Med.* 1983 Mar. 98(3):366-78.

[11] Socin HV, Chanson P, Delemer B, Tabarin A, Rohmer V, Mockel J, Stevenaert A, Beckers A. The changing spectrum of TSH-secreting pituitary adenomas: diagnosis and management in 43 patients. *Eur J Endocrinol* 2003; 148: 433–442.

[12] Tun NN, Beckett G, Zammitt NN, Strachan MW, Seckl JR, Gibb FW. Thyrotropin receptor antibody levels at diagnosis and after thionamide course predict Graves' disease relapse. *Thyroid.* 2016; 26:1004-9.

[13] Ross DS, Burch HB, Cooper DS, Greenlee MC, Laurberg P, Maia AL, Rivkees SA, Samuels M, Sosa JA, Stan MN, Walter MA. American Thyroid Association guidelines for diagnosis and management of hyperthyroidism and other causes of thyrotoxicosis. *Thyroid.* 2016; 26:1343-421.

[14] Bauer DC, Ettinger B, Nevitt MC, Stone KL; Study of Osteoporotic Fractures Research Group. Risk for fracture in women with low serum levels of thyroid-stimulating hormone. *Ann Intern Med.* 2001; 134:561-8.

[15] Summaria V, Salvatori M, Rufini V, Mirk P, Garganese MC, Romani M. Diagnostic imaging in thyrotoxicosis. *Rays* 1999; 24:273–300.

[16] Hari Kumar KV, Pasupuleti V, Jayaraman M, Abhyuday V, Rayudu B R, Modi KD. Role of thyroid Doppler in differential diagnosis of thyrotoxicosis. *Endocr Pract.* 2009 Jan-Feb;15(1):6-9.

[17] Pearce EN. Management of thyrotoxicosis: preconception, pregnancy and the postpartum period. *Endocr Pract.* 2019;25: 62-8.

[18] Perdomo CM, García-Goñi M, Sancho L, J Paricio J, Lozano MD, de la Higuera M, Currás M, Arbizu J, Galofré JC. Evaluation of the role of thyroid scintigraphy in the differential diagnosis of thyrotoxicosis. *Clin Endocrinol (Oxf).* 2021; 94(3):466-472.

[19] Kahaly GJ, Bartalena L, Hegedu L, Leenhardt L, Poppe K, Pearce SH. European Thyroid Association guideline for the management of Graves' hyperthyroidism. *Eur Thyroid J* 2018; 7:167- 86.

[20] Li D, Radulescu A, Shrestha RT, Root M, Karger AB, Killeen AA, Hodges JS, Fan SL, Ferguson A, Garg U, Sokoll LJ, Burmeister LA. Association of biotin ingestion with performance of hormone and nonhormone assays in healthy adults. *JAMA.* 2017; 318:1150-60.

Chapter 6

Subclinical Hyperthyroidism and Its Management

Soumik Goswami and Yashaswi[1,*]

[1]Department of Endocrinology, Nil Ratan Sircar Medical College, Kolkata, India

Abstract

Subclinical hyperthyroidism (SCH) is defined as decreased serum thyroid-stimulating hormone (TSH) with normal serum thyroxine (T4) and triiodothyronine (T3) concentrations. The causes for SCH are similar to those for overt hyperthyroidism and include increased endogenous production and release of thyroid hormone (Graves' disease, toxic nodular goiter, or transient thyroiditis) or excessive intake of levothyroxine. The prevalence of SCH ranges from 0.7-1.8%, with a higher prevalence seen in iodine-deficient areas. The natural history of SCH is variable, with some cases progressing to overt hyperthyroidism (more commonly in those with lower TSH levels), while some may revert to normal TSH levels. SCH is associated with an increased risk of cardiovascular disease, osteoporosis, cognitive decline, and dementia in certain high-risk populations. However, all SCH patients do not need active treatment. Serum TSH level, the patient's age, and the presence of risk factors are used to determine the need for treatment of SCH. Treatment modalities used for SCH are the same as overt hyperthyroidism, and its selection depends on the etiology of SCH and the potential risk-benefit associated with the treatment option.

[*] Corresponding Author's Email: yshswi@gmail.com.

In: Understanding and Managing Hyperthyroidism
Editor: Poongkodi Karunakaran
ISBN: 979-8-88697-636-6

Keywords: subclinical hyperthyroidism, cardiovascular risk, bone loss, management, Graves' disease

1. Introduction

Subclinical hyperthyroidism (SCH) is defined as circulating thyrotropin (thyroid-stimulating hormone; TSH) levels below the lower limit of the normal reference range with normal free thyroid hormone levels, thyroxine (T4), and triiodothyronine (T3). The diagnosis is primarily biochemical because the signs and symptoms of subclinical hyperthyroidism are nonspecific and variable. Because of this, it is essential to define the normal range of TSH to identify patients with SCH. Current assays can detect TSH levels as low as 0.01 mIU/l. However, the normal TSH reference range varies based on the assay used in the laboratory. Commonly used TSH immunometric assays use monoclonal antibodies that differ in specificity and, therefore, may have different normal reference ranges. TSH values also vary based on other factors like age, gender, race, ethnicity, BMI, and iodine status. TSH levels are higher in women, obese, and older populations. It is lower in non-Hispanic African Americans. Because of these factors, it is difficult to define a universal reference range for TSH. The third National Health and Nutrition Examination Survey (NHANES III) established the normal reference range for serum TSH as 0.45 to 4.5 μIU/mL [1]. Based on this, SCH is usually defined as TSH < 0.4 μIU/mL with normal free T4 and T3. Furthermore, SCH patients are classified based on the degree of TSH suppression - SCH with low but detectable TSH (grade 1 or mild) with TSH between 0.1 to 0.4 mIU/L and SCH with suppressed TSH (grade 2 or severe) with TSH < 0.1 mIU/L [2, 3].

2. Prevalence of Subclinical Hyperthyroidism

The prevalence of SCH varies among different populations and is highly dependent on the iodine status. The prevalence of overt hyperthyroidism ranges from 0.7 to 1.8% in iodine-sufficient populations to 2 to 15% in persons with iodine deficiency. It also depends on the TSH assay and cut-off used to define SCH [4]. The Whickham survey, which was conducted before ultrasensitive TSH assays were available, showed the prevalence of SCH (defined as a serum TSH concentration < 0.5 mIU/liter) to be 10% in women but 0% in men [5]. In the NHANES III study, the prevalence of SCH was 0.7% when the TSH cut-off was taken as < 0.1 mIU/Litre, and it reached 3.2% with a TSH cut-off of < 0.4 mIU/liter [1]. In an epidemiological study from Southern India, subclinical and overt hyperthyroidism were present in 1.6% and 1.3% of subjects respectively participating in a community survey [6].

3. Causes of Subclinical Hyperthyroidism

The causes of subclinical hyperthyroidism are the same as those of overt hyperthyroidism. Exogenous causes remain the most common cause of SCH and includes excessive intake of levothyroxine, liothyronine, or desiccated thyroid, intentionally as in the case of patients with follicular cell thyroid cancer, or unintentionally due to overtreatment of hypothyroidism or surreptitiously as in factitious thyrotoxicosis, Among endogenous causes, while Graves' Disease is the most common cause of SCH in younger patients, Toxic Adenoma and Toxic Multinodular Goitre are relatively more common in older patients and iodine-deficient populations.

SCH can also be transient as in the case of subacute, silent, or postpartum thyroiditis. Transient suppression of TSH is also seen after radioiodine ablation of the thyroid in overt hyperthyroidism. TSH suppression may last up to 3-6 months in these cases.

Other causes of TSH suppression must be excluded before classifying it as SCH. These include non-thyroidal illness, psychiatric conditions (depression), drugs like dopamine and glucocorticoids, and secondary hypothyroidism. Pregnancy is also associated with suppressed TSH. This is due to elevated human chorionic gonadotropin level, which because of its homology to TSH, act on TSH receptors increasing thyroid hormone levels and thereby suppressing TSH levels. Excessive iodine intake can also suppress TSH levels, especially in those with underlying thyroid disease [7].

4. Clinical Consequences of Subclinical Hyperthyroidism

4.1. Progression to Overt Hyperthyroidism

Subclinical Hyperthyroidism has a variable evolution. Patients may have stable thyroid dysfunction, progress to overt hyperthyroidism, or revert to euthyroidism over time. The best parameter determining the risk of progression to overt hyperthyroidism is serum TSH level. Patients with TSH < 0.1mIU/L are more likely to progress to overt hyperthyroidism. A large retrospective study showed that 20% of patients with grade 2 SCH progressed to overt hyperthyroidism compared to only 6.8% with grade 1 SCH during seven years of follow-up [8]. Up to 50% of patients with grade 1 SCH can revert to euthyroid status with long-term follow-up.

4.2. Cardiovascular Effects

Thyroid hormones exert important actions on the cardiovascular system. The effects of thyroid hormones on the cardiovascular system are complex and multiple and include genomic and non-genomic effects. While the impact of overt hyperthyroidism on cardiovascular health is commonly known, SCH may also adversely affect cardiac function and morphology.

SCH is associated with atrial arrhythmias, most commonly sinus tachycardia and atrial fibrillation (AF). Atrial and ventricular premature beats and increased heart rate variability are also seen in patients with SCH [7]. Sawin et al., conducted a study in the older population which showed that 28% of patients with subclinical hyperthyroidism developed AF as compared to 11% of those with normal thyroid function [9]. Though AF is more common in older patients, the relative risk of SCH causing AF is higher in younger populations due to the presence of other causes of AF in older populations.

SCH causes an increase in left ventricular mass and left atrial size leading to diastolic dysfunction and impaired systolic function during exercise and hence, impaired exercise tolerance. All these effects on cardiac function increase the risk of heart failure (HF) or worsening of existing heart failure in patients with SCH. A multicentre study conducted on over 25,000 patients found that the risk of HF was increased in subjects with subclinical thyroid dysfunction. The hazard ratio increased from 1.31 in those with TSH 0.10–

0.44 to 1.94 with TSH < 0.10mUI/l after adjustments for other cardiovascular risk factors [10].

The relationship between SCH and stroke is less well-defined. The increased risk of stroke in SCH patients, as seen in certain studies, may be related to the increased prevalence of atrial fibrillation and alterations in coagulation parameters [11].

Several studies have tried to address the association between subclinical hyperthyroidism and all-cause mortality. In a systematic review of more than 50,000 individuals with a median follow-up of 8.8 years, the overall hazard ratios (HRs) for those with SCH compared with euthyroid patients were 1.24 for total mortality, 1.29 for coronary heart disease mortality, 1.21 for coronary heart disease events, and 1.68 for incident atrial fibrillation [12]. SCH was also found to be associated with increased mortality in a population-based study of 5,816 adults. Two other meta-analyses assessing the risk of cardiovascular and all-cause mortality in patients with SCH did not find a link between SCH and mortality [13], [14].

These data, taken together, suggest that the association between cardiovascular morbidity and mortality and subclinical hyperthyroidism might be significant, particularly in the older population.

4.3. Bone Loss

Thyroid hormones act on the bone to increase osteoclastic activity leading to increased bone resorption. This effect is more prominent on cortical bone as compared to trabecular bone. Overt hyperthyroidism is associated with an increased risk of osteoporosis and fractures.

The effect of subclinical hyperthyroidism on bone is not definite and various studies have shown conflicting results. Two large meta-analyses involving patients with exogenous subclinical hyperthyroidism due to TSH suppressive doses of L-thyroxine showed a decrease in bone mineral density (BMD) in postmenopausal women but not in premenopausal women and in men [15]. Another recent meta-analysis including over 70,000 patients with SCH found that SCH was associated with increased risk of hip fractures and any fractures, especially in those with suppressed TSH levels of < 0.1mIU/L and those with endogenous causes of SCH [7].

4.4. Dementia

SCH has been found to be associated with impaired cognition or increased risk of dementia in some studies but the association is not yet definitive. The risk of Alzheimer's Disease and vascular dementia have also been found to be higher in patients with severe SCH [7]. In contrast, a cross-sectional study on 295 patients with subclinical thyroid dysfunction did not show any association between subclinical hyperthyroidism and depression, anxiety, or cognitive function [16].

5. Evaluation

Patients presenting with low TSH and normal free thyroid hormone levels should undergo repeat thyroid function testing, including TSH and free/total T3 and T4, in the next 3-6 months to confirm the diagnosis of SCH and to rule out transient causes of SCH. If biotin-streptavidin assays are being used, biotin supplements should be withheld for at least 2 days before undergoing thyroid function testing since they can interfere with these assays. Once the diagnosis of SCH is biochemically confirmed, other tests need to be done to determine the etiology, as in cases of overt hyperthyroidism. TSH receptor antibody is indicated if Graves' Disease is suspected. Elevated Thyrotropin receptor antibody (TRAb) levels are virtually diagnostic of Graves' Disease, though they may be negative in milder forms of the disease. Hence, a negative test does not rule out Graves' disease diagnosis. In cases where an exogenous cause is suspected, serum thyroglobulin levels are helpful in confirming the diagnosis. In patients where the cause for SCH is exogenous, thyroglobulin levels will be suppressed, while they will be elevated in all cases of endogenous SCH. If excessive iodine intake is suspected as a cause of suppressed TSH levels, 24-hour urinary iodine excretion should be assessed.

Various imaging modalities can also be useful in diagnosing the etiology of SCH and also in guiding treatment. Thyroid scintigraphy is helpful in assessing thyroid gland activity and hence, the underlying cause. There will be decreased uptake in cases of thyroiditis and exogenous thyroid hormone intake, diffusely increased uptake in Graves' Disease patients, and focal area(s) of uptake in cases of toxic multinodular goiter and toxic adenoma. European Thyroid Association (ETA) recommends that scintigraphy be performed in nodular goiters with grade 2 SCH to guide clinicians in the choice of treatment [3]. Ultrasonography with doppler study is recommended in patients with nodular goiter. There will be increased thyroidal blood flow on the doppler study in patients with Graves' disease while it will be decreased in cases of thyroiditis.

Besides evaluating for the underlying etiology of SCH, patients also need to be evaluated for the systemic adverse effects associated with this condition. Electrocardiogram (ECG), echocardiography, and Holter monitoring are recommended by ETA in selected patients with Grade 2 SCH to assess cardiac rhythm and function [3]. Bone mineral density assessment is also needed in selected patients with grade 2 SCH (post-menopausal women, men > 65 years, and those with other risk factors for osteoporosis).

6. Treatment

Once persistently low TSH is confirmed on repeat testing, the decision to treat SCH depends on TSH level, age of the patient, and presence of co-morbidities.

ATA guidelines recommend that SCH with TSH levels < 0.1mIU/L should be treated in all patients aged > 65 years and in patients less than 65 years of age with co-morbidities (osteoporosis, heart disease and postmenopausal women not on estrogens or bisphosphonates) or hyperthyroid symptoms. Treatment can be considered in these same groups of patients if TSH is between 0.1 and 0.4 mIU/L. For asymptomatic patients aged < 65 years and with TSH levels between 0.1-0.4 mIU/L, treatment is not recommended. These patients should be monitored with thyroid function testing every 6-12 months or if symptoms develop [2].

Similar guidelines have also been proposed by ETA which recommend treatment for older patients (> 65 years) with grade 2 SCH and recommend consideration of treatment in grade 1 SCH with co-morbidities including the presence of heart disease, diabetes, renal failure, previous stroke, or transient ischaemic attack, left atrial dilatation, increased risk factors for stroke, HF, CHD, valvular heart disease, and coronary or peripheral arterial disease. Younger patients may be treated if they have Grade 2 SCH with symptoms or TSH receptor Antibody positivity or co-morbidities [3].

The treatment modality selected for patients with SCH is like those for overt hyperthyroid patients and depends on factors like etiology, size of the goiter, and age. In older patients, where toxic multinodular goiter is a common cause, radioiodine ablation may be preferred. Pre-treatment with antithyroid drugs may not be needed in these patients since the risk of exacerbation of hyperthyroidism with radioiodine is low. Low-dose antithyroid drugs can also be used in these patients. Surgery is usually considered only in patients with large goiters causing obstructive symptoms or in patients having a risk of malignancy. In younger patients, Graves' disease is a common cause. Low dose antithyroid drugs (carbimazole 5 to 10 mg) are the preferred mode of treatment in such patients. Low dose antithyroid drugs are also preferred in Graves' disease patients aged > 65 years since the likelihood of remission is high in these patients. Some patients with Graves' disease and SCH remit spontaneously. Therefore, observation with close follow-up may also be a reasonable course, especially in younger patients [3, 7, 17].

The goal of treatment in individuals with SCH is the normalization of serum thyroid function to achieve a euthyroid state in order to reduce the adverse effects of SCH.

Conclusion

Table 1. Recommendations for management of subclinical hyperthyroidism references

		TSH < 0.1mIU/L		**TSH 0.1-0.4mIU/L**	
		ATA	**ETA**	**ATA**	**ETA**
Age > 65 years	Co-morbidities	Treat*	Treat#	Consider Treating*	Treat#
	Symptomatic	Treat	Treat	Consider Treating	Consider Treating
	Asymptomatic	Treat	Treat	Consider Treating	Consider Treating
Age < 65 years	Co-morbidities	Treat*	Treat#	Consider Treating*	Consider Treating#
	Symptomatic	Treat	Consider treating$	Consider Treating	Consider Treating
	Asymptomatic	Consider Treating	Consider treating$	Observe	Observe

*: Heart Disease, Osteoporosis, post-menopausal (not on bisphosphonates or estrogens).

#: heart disease, diabetes, renal failure, previous stroke or transient ischaemic attack, left atrial dilatation, increased risk factors for stroke, HF, CHD, valvular heart disease, and coronary or peripheral arterial disease.

$: TSH- Receptor Antibody positive or increased uptake on radioiodine scan.

Though Subclinical Hyperthyroidism is a biochemical diagnosis with variable clinical presentation, it is not always a benign condition. SCH is associated with adverse effects on cardiovascular and bone health, especially in older populations and in those with more severe TSH suppression. Hence, these patients need to be evaluated further to determine the cause of SCH and the need for further treatment.

References

[1] Hollowell J. G., Staehling N. W., Flanders W. D., Hannon W. H., Gunter E. W., Spencer C. A., & Braverman L. E. Serum TSH, T_4, and Thyroid Antibodies in the United States Population (1988 to 1994): National Health and Nutrition Examination Survey (NHANES III). *The Journal of Clinical Endocrinology & Metabolism.* 2002 Feb;87(2):489–99.

[2] Ross D S, Burch H B, Cooper D S, Greenlee M C, Laurberg P, Maia A L, Rivkees S A, Samuels M, Sosa J A, Stan M N, Walter M A. 2016 American Thyroid Association Guidelines for Diagnosis and Management of Hyperthyroidism and Other Causes of Thyrotoxicosis. *Thyroid.* 2016 Oct 1;26(10):1343–421.

[3] Biondi B, Bartalena L, Cooper D S, Hegedüs L, Laurberg P, Kahaly G J. The 2015 European Thyroid Association Guidelines on Diagnosis and Treatment of Endogenous Subclinical Hyperthyroidism. *European Thyroid Journal.* 2015;4(3): 149–63.

[4] Biondi B, Cooper D S. Subclinical Hyperthyroidism. Solomon C G, editor. *New England Journal of Medicine [Internet].* 2018 Jun 21;378(25):2411–9. Available from: http://www.nejm.org/doi/10.1056/NEJMcp1709318.

[5] Vanderpump M P, Tunbridge W M, French J M, Appleton D, Bates D, Clark F, Grimley Evans J, Hasan D M, Rodgers H, Tunbridge F. The incidence of thyroid disorders in the community: a twenty-year follow-up of the Whickham Survey. *Clinical Endocrinology.* 1995 Jul;43(1):55–68.

[6] Unnikrishnan A, Menon U. Thyroid disorders in India: An epidemiological perspective. *Indian Journal of Endocrinology and Metabolism.* 2011;15(6):78.

[7] Tsai K, Leung A M. *Subclinical Hyperthyroidism: A Review of the Clinical Literature.* Vol. 27, Endocrine Practice. Elsevier B.V.; 2021. p. 254–60.

[8] Das G, Ojewuyi T A, Baglioni P, Geen J, Premawardhana L D, Okosieme O E. Serum thyrotrophin at baseline predicts the natural course of subclinical hyperthyroidism. *Clinical Endocrinology.* 2012 Jul;77(1):146–51.

[9] Sawin C T, Geller A, Wolf PA, Belanger AJ, Baker E, Bacharach P, Wilson PW, Benjamin EJ, D'Agostino R B. Low Serum Thyrotropin Concentrations as a Risk Factor for Atrial Fibrillation in Older Persons. *New England Journal of Medicine.* 1994 Nov 10;331(19):1249–52.

[10] Gencer B, Collet T H, Virgini V, Bauer D C, Gussekloo J, Cappola A R, Nanchen D, den Elzen W P, Balmer P, Luben R N, Iacoviello M, Triggiani V, Cornuz J, Newman A B, Khaw K T, Jukema J W, Westendorp R G, Vittinghoff E, Aujesky D, Rodondi N. Subclinical Thyroid Dysfunction and the Risk of Heart Failure Events. *Circulation.* 2012 Aug 28;126(9):1040–9.

[11] Delitala A P. *Subclinical Hyperthyroidism and the Cardiovascular Disease.* Vol. 49, Hormone and Metabolic Research. Georg Thieme Verlag; 2017. p. 723–31.

[12] Collet T H, Gussekloo J, Bauer D C, den Elzen W P, Cappola A R, Balmer P, Iervasi G, Åsvold B O, Sgarbi J A, Völzke H, Gencer B, Maciel R M, Molinaro S, Bremner A, Luben R N, Maisonneuve P, Cornuz J, Newman A B, Khaw K T, Westendorp R G, Franklyn J A, Vittinghoff E, Walsh J P, Rodondi N. Subclinical Hyperthyroidism and the Risk of Coronary Heart Disease and Mortality. *Archives of Internal Medicine.* 2012 May 28;172(10).

[13] Singh S, Duggal J, Molnar J, Maldonado F, Barsano C P, Arora R. Impact of subclinical thyroid disorders on coronary heart disease, cardiovascular and all-cause mortality: A meta-analysis. *International Journal of Cardiology.* 2008 Mar;125 (1):41–8.

[14] Völzke H, Schwahn C, Wallaschofski H, Dörr M. The Association of Thyroid Dysfunction with All-Cause and Circulatory Mortality: Is There a Causal Relationship? *The Journal of Clinical Endocrinology & Metabolism.* 2007 Jul 1;92(7):2421–9.

[15] Hoogendoorn E H, den Heijer M, van Dijk A P J, Hermus A R. Subclinical hyperthyroidism: To treat or not to treat? Vol. 80, *Postgraduate Medical Journal.* 2004. p. 394–8.

[16] Palacios S S, Pascual-Corrales E, Galofre JC. Management of subclinical hyperthyroidism. Vol. 10, *International Journal of Endocrinology and Metabolism.* 2012. p. 490–6.

[17] Holick M F, Binkley N C, Bischoff-Ferrari H A, Gordon C M, Hanley D A, Heaney R P, Murad M H, Weaver C M. Evaluation, treatment, and prevention of vitamin D deficiency: An endocrine society clinical practice guideline. Vol. 96, *Journal of Clinical Endocrinology and Metabolism.* 2011. p. 1911–30.

Chapter 7

Medical Management of Hyperthyroidism

Poongkodi Karunakaran[1,2,3*]
Pattanam Velappan Dhanapal[4]
Vijayakumar Krishnaswamy[4]
Sureshkanna Singaram[4]
and Felix Jebasingh[5]
[1]Endocrine Surgery Unit, Government Mohan Kumaramangalam Medical College, Salem, India
[2]Department of Endocrine Surgery, Madras Medical College, Chennai, India
[3]The Tamilnadu Dr. MGR Medical University, Chennai, India
[4]Government Mohan Kumaramangalam Medical College, Salem, Tamilnadu, India
[5]Christian Medical College, Vellore, Tamilnadu, India

Abstract

Medical management is the mainstay of treatment for hyperthyroidism and it is the initial treatment modality for patients requiring definitive therapeutic options, either radioactive iodine or surgery. Thionamides are the first line of drugs. Alternative drugs are used for controlling hyperthyroidism wherein thionamides cannot be used. Similarly, adjuvant therapy combined with thionamides may be required for rapid and effective control of hyperthyroidism in special clinical scenarios. The choice of drug is individualized considering underlying etiology, current symptoms, long-term risks, adverse effects, cost-effectiveness, and patient's preferences. This chapter describes the mechanism of action, clinical indications, and side effects of various thyroid inhibitors including future targeted therapies.

* Corresponding Author's Email: poongkodithesurgeon@gmail.com

In: Understanding and Managing Hyperthyroidism
Editor: Poongkodi Karunakaran
ISBN: 979-8-88697-636-6

Keywords: antithyroid drug, thionamides, non-thionamide antithyroid drugs, monoclonal antibodies, and small-molecule ligands

Introduction

Hyperthyroidism is defined as increased synthesis and secretion of thyroid hormone by the thyroid gland per se [1]. Whereas, thyrotoxicosis is a constellation of signs and symptoms caused by excessive circulating thyroid hormone concentrations [2]. The ideal treatment of hyperthyroidism should be directed at its etiology. The common causes of hyperthyroidism include Graves' disease (GD), toxic multinodular goiter (TMNG) and toxic adenoma (TA). The etiology of these clinical entities remains elusive. Hence, the therapeutic objectives of hyperthyroidism are aimed at 1) reduction of thyroid hormone concentrations to achieve euthyroidism 2) maintenance of stable euthyroid status, 2) control of disease manifestations 3) reduce morbidity and 4) cost-effectiveness. The currently available therapeutic options are antithyroid medications, radioactive iodine (RAI) therapy and total thyroidectomy. All three treatment modalities have merits and demerits. However, a recent non-randomized trial reported impaired quality of life after RAI therapy in the long term compared to surgery or medical management of Graves' hyperthyroidism [3]. Medical management of hyperthyroidism is the initial treatment modality, but definitive therapeutic options include either RAI ablation or surgical removal of thyroid gland. The choice of therapy is influenced by many factors such as intolerance or non-compliance to antithyroid drugs, large volume goiter, presence of pressure symptoms, retrosternal extension, suspicion of malignancy, pregnancy, thyroid eye disease, and cardiotoxicity. The availability of nuclear medicine infrastructure, surgical expertise, geographical biases, clinician and patient's preferences can impact the therapeutic decision [4, 5]. This chapter discusses the medical management of hyperthyroidism.

Medical management of hyperthyroidism aims to lower the functional capacity of the hyperactive thyroid gland with thyroid inhibitors. Thyroid inhibitors are classified as agents that 1) inhibit or interfere with thyroid hormone synthesis and release, 2) modify tissue responsiveness to thyroid hormones, and 3) destroy the thyroid gland with radiation [6]. Conventionally, only drugs that inhibit thyroid hormone biosynthesis are known as antithyroid drugs (ATDs). In general, thionamides are referred as an antithyroid drug while others are grouped under non-thionamide antithyroid drugs (NTAD) [7].

Briefly, thyroid hormone biosynthesis consists of iodide trapping against the 100-fold concentration gradient by sodium-iodide symporter (NIS) of thyroid follicular cells, thyroperoxidase-enzyme complex mediated iodide oxidation, and organification of iodotyrosyl residues at the thyroglobulin-colloidal interface, coupling reaction of mono-iodothyronine and di-iodothyronine to form 3,5,3' tri-iodothyronine (T3) and 3, 5, 3', 5' tetraiodothyronine (T4), and finally, proteolysis and secretion of thyroid hormones into the circulation. The ratio of T4 to T3 bound to thyroglobulin is 13:1 and hence, T4 is predominant form released into the circulation. T4 is converted to biologically active T3 by mono-deiodination of the outer ring by 5' deiodinase (5'DI) in the peripheral tissues [8]. T3 is 99.7% protein bound and 0.3% is free form with plasma half-life of 1 day. Whereas, T4 is more tightly protein bound (99.97%) with a longer plasma half-life of 7 days and acts as a prohormone. The half-lives are shortened in hyperthyroidism due to higher metabolic rate. We shall consider the mechanism of action, indications and side effect profile of thyroid inhibitors in detail.

Classification of Thyroid Inhibitors

Thionamides or Antithyroid Drugs (ATD)

Thionamides are heterocyclic compounds that contain the thioureylene group having antithyroid activity. Three available drugs are carbimazole (1-methyl-2-thio-3 carbethoxy-imidazole), methimazole (1-methyl 2-mercaptoimidazole; MMI), and propylthiouracil (6-propyl-2-thiouracil; PTU). Carbimazole is a prodrug of methimazole, and about 10 mg of carbimazole yields 6 mg of MMI by in vivo metabolism. Carbimazole is widely used in the United Kingdom whereas MMI is widely used in the United States and Japan. Both carbimazole and MMI are available in India and a few other countries.

Pharmacodynamics

Thionamides exert intrathyroidal and extrathyroidal action. The major intrathyroidal action is competitive inhibition of thyroperoxidase-mediated iodide oxidation and organification, and inhibition of peroxidase-catalyzed coupling reaction. Thionamides possibly alter thyroglobulin structure and inhibit thyroglobulin biosynthesis as well. ATDs do not interfere with iodide trapping. They do not modify T3 or T4 actions on peripheral tissues or the pituitary. Since thionamides inhibit the synthesis of new hormones and do not interfere with the release of preformed hormones, T3 and T4 concentrations begin to decline when intrathyroidal stores are depleted, often requiring 3 to 4 weeks. In addition, PTU but not MMI inhibits the conversion of T4 to T3 in the peripheral tissues. PTU inactivates type I T4-deiodinase by covalently binding to the enzyme through a selenosulfide bond. Hence, PTU rapidly decreases the biologically active T3 levels and is helpful in life-threatening thyroid storms. However, more rapid normalization of T4 and T3 to euthyroid levels is achieved with thioimidazoles compared to PTU. Thionamides are reported to have immunosuppressive actions. Decline in serum concentrations of antithyroid antibodies and TSH receptor antibodies (TSHR-Ab) and changes in T-cell subsets have been reported in patients receiving ATDs. Indeed, MMI has been shown to decrease intrathyroidal activated T cells.

Pharmacokinetics

MMI is almost completely absorbed from the gastrointestinal tract and reaches peak serum concentrations of 300 mg/ml within 1-2 hours after an oral dose of 15 mg. The plasma half-life of MMI is 6 to 8 hours and is unaltered in thyrotoxicosis. Similarly, drug clearance is unaltered in thyrotoxicosis but may slow in patients with hepatic disease. Being lipid soluble and non-protein bound, MMI freely cross membranes including placenta and breast epithelium. MMI rapidly accumulates in the thyroid gland and reaches an intrathyroidal concentration of 500 to 2000 ng/g. Intrathyroidal turnover of MMI is slow and accounts for the longer duration of action. An oral dose of 30 mg of MMI exerts anti-thyroid activity for longer than 24 hours. Given the intrathyroidal accumulation and longer duration of action, a single daily dose of MMI is effective despite the short half-life. For the same reason, MMI is ten-fold more potent than PTU. Little is known about the fate of MMI or its metabolic products, and little MMI is excreted in the urine. MMI is a hepatic enzyme inducer and higher doses of Glucocorticoids may be required in hyperthyroid patients with Thyroid Eye Disease (TED). The American Thyroid Association has recommended initial dosing of MMI based on the baseline free T4 levels. An oral daily dose of MMI 5-10 mg, 10-20 mg and 30-40 mg is given for free T4 levels of 2-3 ng/dL, 3-4 ng/dL, and 4-6 ng/dL respectively above the normal upper limit (2 ng/dL). Thyroid profile is monitored, and dosage is titrated every 4-6 weeks. On achieving euthyroid status, a lower maintenance dose is employed, otherwise, hypothyroidism may ensue. It is imperative to maintain normal or upper normal limits of thyroid hormones in hyperthyroid patients with TED, as hypothyroidism can worsen TED.

In contrast, PTU is rapidly absorbed and reaches peak serum concentrations of about 3 mg/mL within an hour after ingestion. But the bioavailability of PTU is only 50-80% due to high first-pass metabolism in the liver. PTU has a shorter half-life of 1.5 hours. PTU is accumulated by the thyroid gland, and an oral dose of 100 mg of PTU can decrease iodine organification by 60% for 7 to 8 hours. Given the shorter half-life and duration of action, PTU is administered more frequently every 8 hours. Being tightly protein-bound (80-90%) and ionized at physiological pH, PTU does not cross the membranes freely. PTU undergoes glucuronide conjugation in the liver and is excreted in the urine. A daily oral dose of 300 mg PTU is recommended initially in three divided doses. The dosage and frequency may be reduced over time.

Adverse Effects

Fever, urticaria, maculopapular rash and arthralgia occurs in 1-5% of the patients on MMI. Mild rash resolves spontaneously despite the continuation of the drug or may require anti-histamines. Severe allergic reaction needs drug discontinuation. Other minor side effects include nausea, alteration of taste and smell, and arthritis. Agranulocytosis is rare (0.2 to 0.5%) but life-threatening, particularly in elderly patients receiving MMI of more than 40 mg per day. Agranulocytosis is defined as a granulocyte count of fewer than 250 cells per cubic mm and often heralds as pharyngitis with gram-negative organisms. Patients should be educated to seek immediate medical attention if symptoms develop. Confirmation with complete blood count (CBC), prompt cessation of antithyroid drug, appropriate antibiotics, and treatment with Granulocyte-Colony Stimulating factors (G-CSF) is life-saving. As the cross-reactivity between MMI and PTU is 50%, switching drugs should not be attempted. Mild granulocytopenia (Granulocyte count less than 1500 cells per cubic mm) occurs in 10% of untreated thyrotoxic patients and in normal African patients. Similarly, aplastic anemia characterized by hematocrit > 30% and low platelet count needs prompt attention. Hence, a baseline CBC is recommended for all patients before initiating ATD and periodic monitoring in selective patients. Hepatotoxicity is another serious adverse effect of ATDs. PTU-induced fulminant hepatitis is rare but fatal and may need liver transplantation. African American children are at a higher risk. A PTU dose of 300 mg daily can increase the risk of liver failure and is common in the first 4-months after starting therapy. Patients should be educated about the warning signs and to discontinue the drug if they develop malaise, jaundice, dark urine, and grey-colored stools. A few studies support MMI switching in these patients as MMI causes a different type of liver injury. MMI may cause cholestatic hepatitis with hyperbilirubinemia and bile duct stasis, but the hepatocellular architecture remains preserved. Vasculitis or drug induced lupus like syndrome is associated with PTC and rarely with MMI. Glucocorticoid therapy is given for symptomatic patients with myeloperoxidase-ANCA-related vasculitis and severe cases may require immunosuppressants like cyclophosphamides. Similarly, antithyroid arthritis syndrome occurs in 1-2% of ANCA-negative patients and resolves with the discontinuation of drugs. These patients should be immediately started on beta-adrenergic blockers or inorganic iodide, or an alternative drug regimen until definitive treatment with surgery or RAI therapy is feasible. PTU-induced hypoprothrombinemia, MMI-induced hypoglycemia due to insulin autoimmune syndrome, MMI-induced pancreatitis are rarer but serious side effects. Importantly, being lipid-soluble and little protein bound, MMI can freely cross placental membranes and cause aplasia cutis, or methimazole embryopathy characterized by choanal atresia or esophageal atresia. In contrast, a little PTU crosses the membranes freely as PTU is highly protein-bound and ionized at physiological pH. Hence, PTU is the preferred drug for treating hyperthyroidism during the first trimester of pregnancy and in nursing mothers.

Clinical Uses

ATD is the drug of choice for the long-term treatment of hyperthyroidism in adults, adolescents and children [9]. ATDs are used initially for preoperative preparation to achieve euthyroid status or prior to RAI therapy to blunt thyroid hormone excursions and prevent thyroid storms. However, PTU can exert a radioprotective effect by neutralizing iodinated free radicals, thereby decreasing the efficacy of subsequent RAI therapy. ATD can be given for a period of 18 to 24 months and tapered slowly before cessation or switched to definitive treatment if the disease persists. ATDs induce remission in 30-50% of Graves' disease (GD) patients. Remission is defined as remaining biochemically euthyroid after one year of cessation of antithyroid treatment. Recurrence is not uncommon and can occur at any time but recurs commonly in the first year after remission. Predictors of remission include female gender, milder disease, small goiter, and low TSHR-Ab. Predictors of recurrence include large volume goiter, the severity of the disease, high baseline T3 and T4, high titers of antithyroid antibodies, and TSHR-Ab. Higher potency, better tolerability, better pharmacological profile, and improved adherence with once-daily dosing make MMI the drug of choice. ATA and US Food and Drug Administration recommend MMI as the first-line therapy for the treatment of hyperthyroidism. PTU was the preferred drug until a black box warning was issued as it can cause fatal hepatitis. PTU is currently reserved for special situations including life-threatening thyroid storm, first-trimester of pregnancy and in nursing mothers, and intolerance to MMI. Patient education about the adverse effects is mandatory before initiating treatment. The most important disadvantage of ATD is poor compliance.

Iodine and Iodides

Iodine is reduced to iodide in the intestine. Hence, the actions of iodine and iodide are identical. Iodine is a constituent of thyroid hormones and affects all facets of thyroid function. The most important action of iodine is thyroid constipation. In therapeutic doses of 6 mg per day, iodide blocks thyroid hormone release by halting endocytosis of colloid and proteolysis of thyroglobulin. T3 and T4 levels decline rapidly within 2 to 7 days, making iodides the fastest-acting thyroid inhibitor and valuable in the treatment of thyroid storm. However, the larger stores of intraglandular iodine can delay the onset of action of thionamides as well as prevent treatment with RAI for several weeks. Hence, iodides are given after initiating therapy with thionamides and are avoided if contemplating RAI therapy. Excessive iodine inhibits its own transport into the thyroid follicular cells and can cause acute inhibition of organification by altering the redox potential, thereby decreasing T3 and T4 synthesis which is known as Wolff-Chaikoff's effect. One proposed mechanism is the formation of organic iodocompounds called iodohexadecanal within the thyroid gland, which exerts inhibitory effects on adenylate cyclase, NADPH oxidase, and thyroperoxidase, thereby inhibiting organification and subsequent hormone synthesis [10]. It is possibly an auto-regulatory mechanism to prevent excessive hormone synthesis when iodine intake is high. In addition, iodides decrease vascularity, size, and fragility of the hyperplastic thyroid gland, improving its handling during surgery. However, thyroid inhibition escapes within 2-6 weeks, worsening thyrotoxicosis in an already iodine-enriched environment. Hence, iodides should be administered only for a short duration in patients pre-treated with thionamides. Two drops of a saturated solution of potassium iodide (35-50 mg iodide/drop) 3 times a day or a drop of Lugol's iodine (8 mg/drop) 3 times a day is given 10 days prior to surgery. Collosol and colloid iodine are other preparations available. In nuclear outbreaks, prophylactic potassium iodide can protect the gland from radiation-induced injury. Acute reaction to iodides is uncommon and resolves with discontinuation. Chronic overdose can result in iodism characterized by conjunctivitis, rhinorrhea, salivation, drug fever or rarely anaphylactoid reactions. Long-term use in pregnant and lactating mothers can cause fetal or infantile goiter and hypothyroidism.

Radioactive Iodine

131-I is the radioactive isotope of iodine used for the definitive treatment of hyperthyroidism. Beta rays emitted by 131-I have therapeutic potential. The physical half-life of beta rays is 8 days and penetration power ranges from 400-2000 μm. About 15-20 millicurie of 131-I administered orally as tablet or solution of sodium is rapidly absorbed. RAI is trapped by the thyroid gland and incorporated into the colloid. Beta rays of 131-I destroys the thyroid gland from within the follicles. A low dose of 5-10 millicurie has a higher failure rate and recurrence, while higher dose is associated with progressive hypothyroidism. Pre-treatment with thionamides reduces radiation-induced thyroiditis but can reduce the efficacy of subsequent RAI therapy [6]. Similarly, iodides have shown mixed success after RAI therapy, particularly in recurrent thyrotoxicosis. Potassium iodide given one week after RAI therapy do not interfere with radioiodine thyroidal uptake. Iodides combined with MMI can rapidly decrease thyroid hormone levels. Moreover, the escape from the Wolff-Chaikoff's effect is less likely after RAI therapy and hypothyroidism develops quickly. RAI therapy is contraindicated in pregnant and nursing mothers as it can destroy the fetal thyroid. Also, given the doubt of carcinogenesis and genetic damage, RAI is avoided in children.

Iodinated Oral Cholecystography Agents

Iodinated triiodoaniline derivatives including sodium iopanoate (Telepaque) and sodium ipodate (Oragrafin) are radiographic contrast agents used for cholecystography. They inhibit peripheral T4 to T3 conversion, acutely lowering T3 levels by inhibiting T4-deiodinase [5, 6]. These iodinated compounds per se and inorganic iodides released from their deiodination can inhibit thyroid hormone synthesis and release. These agents are given orally at 1 g per day in T4 poisoning, thyrotoxic storm, amiodarone-induced thyrotoxicosis and severe neonatal thyrotoxicosis [7].

Anion Inhibitors

Monovalent anions competitively inhibit iodide trapping into the thyroid follicular cells by binding to NIS, due to similar hydrated ion size. Thiocyanate (SCN-), perchlorates (ClO4-) and pertechnetate (TcO4-) are ionic inhibitors available in the decreasing order of potency. Potassium perchlorate can discharge iodine from the thyroid gland, thereby lowering intrathyroidal iodine and hormone synthesis. Perchlorate is used in iodine-induced hyperthyroidism related to amiodarone exposure. Although high-dose thionamide are the first line of drugs in type I amiodarone induced hyperthyroidism (AIT), perchlorates are useful adjunctive as it decreases thyroid iodine uptake and reuptake [7, 11]. The usual dose of potassium perchlorate is 1 g per day in divided doses for 2-6 weeks. Anion inhibitors have severe toxicity profile, and a few cases of fatal aplastic anemia has been reported with perchlorates.

Beta Adrenoceptor Blocking Agents

Manifestations of thyrotoxicosis mimic those of sympathetic overactivity. Beta blockers facilitate rapid symptom relief in thyrotoxicosis and are effective therapeutic adjuncts. They do not affect thyroid function or thyroid hormone synthesis. Beta blockers without intrinsic sympathomimetic activity including metoprolol, propranolol and atenolol are preferred and are often combined with thionamides. ATA recommends beta blockers in elderly patients with symptomatic thyrotoxicosis, patients with resting pulse rate exceeding 90 per minute, and those with cardiovascular complications [9]. Beta blockers are avoided in patients with heart blocks, heart failure, and asthma. Beta blockers may be considered in thyrotoxic patients with heart failure precipitated by atrial fibrillation. However, digitalization often combined with antithrombotic agents is safe in these situations. Propranolol per oral, 160 mg/day or more in divided doses inhibits the peripheral conversion of T4 to T3 and rapidly decreases T3 levels. Intravenous Propranolol 1-2 mg every 6th hour or short-acting intravenous esmolol (50-100 µg/kg/min) along with glucocorticoids and thionamides are used to treat thyroid storms [7, 12]. Beta-blockers are contraindicated in patients with asthma, heart failure, and bradyarrhythmia. Diltiazem, a calcium channel blocker may be considered in these patients for control of tachycardia, severe hypertension, and cardiovascular complications related to thyrotoxic crisis.

Lithium Carbonate

Lithium carbonate is available in two forms. The immediate-release preparation reaches peak serum concentrations in 1-2 hours after oral ingestion, while sustained release lithium carbonate attains peak slowly after 4-5 hours. The plasma half-life is 18-36 hours. Lithium is mostly excreted by the kidney, and its clearance can decrease in renal failure and advancing age. The thyroid concentrates lithium about 3 to 4-fold against the concentration gradient by active transport. The primary mechanism of lithium carbonate is the inhibition of TSH action on cAMP. TSH stimulates all the major steps involved in thyroid hormone synthesis and release. However, the major action of lithium is the inhibition of TSH-mediated thyroid hormone release and can affect hormone synthesis too [7, 13, 14]. There are a few reports of thyroid "escape" from lithium inhibition. Lithium is primarily used for bipolar maniac depressive disorders [15]. Thionamides are the preferred line of drugs for hyperthyroidism management. However, lithium has a role as an alternative drug when thionamides could be used due to intolerance or any contraindication. Lithium is an effective adjunct to RAI therapy in the management of hyperthyroidism. Lithium inhibits iodine release from the thyroid gland without affecting thyroidal iodine uptake, thereby increasing the retention of radioiodine. Thus, lithium increases the efficacy of radioiodine and protects against exacerbations of thyrotoxicosis resulting from preformed hormone release. Studies have shown that RAI-lithium combination therapy can improve the cure rates, quicken the time to cure, and blunt thyroid hormone excursions [16,17]. Similarly, adjunctive lithium may be used in patients with type 1 AIT, who did not respond to conventional high-dose thionamides and glucocorticoids.

The usual dose of lithium is 300-450 mg per oral every 8 hours. Lithium has a narrow therapeutic window, and serum concentration should be maintained at 1 mEq/L. Close monitoring of serum lithium is recommended one week after initiation of therapy or dose titration and monthly thereafter. Lithium toxicity is classified as mild, moderate, and severe. Mild lithium toxicity at 1.5-2 mEq/L causes nausea, vomiting, diarrhea, hand tremor, and drowsiness. Moderate toxicity at 2-2.5 mEq/L causes myoclonic twitches, nystagmus, dysarthria, ataxia, and confusion. Sever toxicity at lithium concentration exceeding 2.5 mEq/L manifest as renal impairment, seizure, coma, and death.

Glucocorticoids

Hydrocortisone and dexamethasone are effective therapeutic adjuncts in hyperthyroidism under special circumstances. The mechanism of action is inhibition of T4 to T3 conversion in peripheral tissues, thereby lowering the biological active T3 levels. This has clinical implications in treating thyroid storm combined with beta-blockers, thionamides, and supportive measures. Intravenous hydrocortisone, 300 mg loading dose followed by 100 mg every 8 hours is given. Alternatively, dexamethasone 8 mg daily may be given. Glucocorticoids are tapered off with improving signs. Similarly, Glucocorticoids can facilitate rapid preoperative preparation of toxic goiter combined with thionamides or beta blockers. Oral or intravenous hydrocortisone 100 mg every 8 hours or alternatively, oral or intravenous dexamethasone 2 mg every 6 hours is given and should be tapered off within 72 hours post-surgery [7]. The high dose-short course treatment regimen of glucocorticoids in hyperthyroidism can cause an acute rise in blood pressure, blood glucose, and suppress the immunological response. This could benefit a subset of patients with adrenal insufficiency, which is not uncommon in hyperthyroidism. Pulsed methylprednisolone is recommended in thyroid eye disease (TED) patients having high clinical activity scores.

Cholestyramine

Cholestyramine is an ion exchange resin. Cholestyramine is a bile acid sequestrant and can interfere with enterohepatic circulation. Both T3 and T4 are steroid hormones that undergo enterohepatic circulation. Both T3 and T4 are concentrated in the liver and undergo glucuronide or sulphate conjugation. The conjugated form and a fraction of free form are secreted in the bile into the intestine. Bacterial deconjugation releases the free thyroid hormone, which is reabsorbed into the circulation, thereby completing enterohepatic circulation. Cholestyramine resin can bind thyroid hormone in the intestine and inhibit reabsorption into the circulation. Adjuvant therapy of cholestyramine in Graves' disease when combined with thionamide can hasten the attainment of euthyroid status compared to thionamide monotherapy [7, 18, 19]. It can be used to rapidly lower T3 and T4 levels, as an alternative therapy when first-line drugs cannot be used in thyroid storm. Cholestyramine use can benefit patients with contrast-induced hyperthyroidism. Oral Cholestyramine 2 grams 2 to 4 times a day is the usual dose. Side effects include bloating, flatulence, and constipation. Cholestyramine can bind concomitantly given drugs and decrease their efficacy.

Future Therapies

Novel therapies targeting the etiopathogenesis of Graves' disease are being developed worldwide. Graves' disease is an autoimmune disorder characterized by persistent unregulated stimulation of thyrotropin receptor (TSHR) on thyrocytes by long-acting stimulatory autoantibodies [20]. Many of the B-cell functions attribute to GD. B-cells are precursors of plasma cells that produce TSHR-Abs. B-cells can act as antigen-presenting cells that initiate the inflammatory cascade and affect cell-mediated immunity by T4-helper cells. Hence, novel medications are directed at B-cell function and TSHR.

Rituximab

Rituximab is a chimeric murine anti-CD20 monoclonal antibody directed against pre-, immature-, mature- and memory-B cells. Rituximab depletes peripheral B cells by inducing apoptosis, antibody-dependent cellular toxicity and complement-mediated lysis. A randomized controlled trial has shown a decline in TSHR-Ab levels in GD patients receiving rituximab compared to the non-rituximab group and hence, the possibility of sustained remission. Rituximab has shown promising results in patients with active Graves's orbitopathy who did not respond to glucocorticoid therapy [21].

Novel Therapies Targeting Thyrotropin Receptors

Two classes of novel medications targeting TSHR are monoclonal antibodies (MAbs) to TSHR, and small-molecule ligands (SMLs) [20, 22].

Thyrotropin Receptor Monoclonal Antibodies

TSHR-Abs are classified as stimulating, blocking, and neutral antibodies based on their actions. Blocking MAbs and inverse agonist MAbs to TSHR are being investigated to treat immune and non-immune hyperthyroidism. KI-70 is a MAb having TSHR antagonist properties. KI-70 can inhibit TSH and TSHR-Ab- mediated receptor activation. It could benefit patients with TSH-secreting pituitary tumors. 5C9 is a MAb having TSHR inverse agonist activity which can exert an inhibitory effect on TSHR activation as well decrease TSHR basal activity. It might benefit patients with non-immune hyperthyroidism harboring TSHR mutations that results in constitutive activation of TSHR and signal transduction cascade.

Small-Molecule Ligands Binding to TSH

SML binding to the transmembrane domain of TSHR inhibits the activation of TSHR. SMLs do not affect TRAb binding to the ectodomain of TSHR. Two types are SML-TSH antagonist and SML TSHR inverse agonists. SML-TSH antagonist including NCGC00242595 inhibit the activation of TSHR and subsequent, TSH mediated upregulation of TPO expression and cAMP production. They could inhibit TSHR signaling mediated by TSHR-Ab. SML TSHR inverse agonists which are being investigated in model cell system could inhibit both the TSH-signaling pathway as well as basal activity. In addition, they could inhibit TSHR-Ab mediated stimulation of TSHR signaling cascade [7].

Conclusion

Thionamide is the drug of choice for the treatment of hyperthyroidism. Beta blocker are effective adjuncts for prompt symptom relief. An alternative line of drugs including iodides, anion inhibitors, iodinated contrast agents and cholestyramine are useful when thionamides cannot be used due to intolerance or contraindication. In special circumstances, alternative drugs are useful adjuvants to facilitate rapid and effective control of hyperthyroidism. Understanding the pharmacological profile and proper patient selection are the key factors in deciding the choice and success of therapy. Novel medications targeting B-cell function and TSHR including rituximab, monoclonal antibodies, and small-molecule ligands are under investigation.

References

[1] de Leo S., Lee S. Y., Braverman L. E. Hyperthyroidism. Vol. 388, *The Lancet.* 2016. p. 906–18.

[2] Franklyn J. A., Boelaert K. Thyrotoxicosis. In: *The Lancet.* 2012. p. 1155–66.

[3] Törring O., Watt T., Sjölin G., Byström K., Abraham-Nordling M., Calissendorff J., Cramon P. K., Filipsson Nyström H., Hallengren B., Holmberg M., Khamisi S., Lantz M., Wallin G. Impaired Quality of Life After Radioiodine Therapy Compared to Antithyroid Drugs or Surgical Treatment for Graves' Hyperthyroidism: A Long-Term Follow-Up with the Thyroid-Related Patient-Reported Outcome Questionnaire and 36-Item Short Form Health Status Survey. *Thyroid.* 2019 Mar 15;29(3):322–31.

[4] Abadin S. S., Cabanillas M. E., Boger M. S., Perrier N. D. Graves' and Plummer's Diseases: Medical and Surgical Management. In: Clark O. H., Duh Q. Y., Kebebew E., Gosnell J. E., Shen Wen T., editors. *Textbook of Endocrine Surgery.* 3rd ed. Philadelphia: The Health Sciences Publisher; 2016.

[5] Cooper D. S. Treatment of thyrotoxicosis. In: Braverman L. E., Cooper D. S., Kopp P., editors. *Werner & Ingbar's The Thyroid: A Fundamental and Clinical Text.* 11th ed. Wolters Kluwer Health; 2021. p. 495–523.

[6] Masters S. B., Rosenthal S. M. Thyroid and Antithyroid Drugs. In: Katzung B. G., Masters S. B., Trevor A. J., editors. *Basic and Clinical Pharmacology.* 12th ed. New Delhi: Tata McGraw Hill Education Private Limited; 2012. p. 681–96.

[7] Suwansaksri N., Preechasuk L., Kunavisarut T. Nonthionamide Drugs for the Treatment of Hyperthyroidism: From Present to Future. *Int J Endocrinol.* 2018;2018:1–10.

[8] Kopp P. A. Thyroid Hormone Synthesis. In: Braverman L. E., Cooper D. S., Kopp P. A., editors. *Werner & Ingbar's The Thyroid: A Fundamental and Clinical Text.* 11th ed. Cooper, David S: Lippincott Williams & Wilkins (LWW); 2021. p. 59–85.

[9] Ross D. S., Burch H. B., Cooper D. S., Greenlee M. C., Laurberg P., Maia A. L., Rivkees S. A., Samuels M., Sosa J. A., Stan M. N., Walter M. A. 2016 American Thyroid Association Guidelines for Diagnosis and Management of Hyperthyroidism and Other Causes of Thyrotoxicosis. *Thyroid.* 2016 Oct;26(10):1343–421.

[10] Dugrillon A. Iodolactones and iodoaldehydes - mediators of iodine in thyroid autoregulation. *Experimental and Clinical Endocrinology & Diabetes.* 2009 Jul 15;104(S 04):41–5.

[11] Merrill E. A. PBPK Model for Radioactive Iodide and Perchlorate Kinetics and Perchlorate-Induced Inhibition of Iodide Uptake in Humans. *Toxicological Sciences*. 2004 Oct 13;83(1):25–43.

[12] Satoh T., Isozaki O., Suzuki A., Wakino S., Iburi T., Tsuboi K., Kanamoto N., Otani H, Furukawa Y, Teramukai S, Akamizu T. 2016 Guidelines for the management of thyroid storm from The Japan Thyroid Association and Japan Endocrine Society (First edition). *Endocr J*. 2016;63(12):1025–64.

[13] Kristensen O., Harrestrup Andersen H., Pallisgaard G. Lithium Carbonate In The Treatment of Thyrotoxicosis. *The Lancet*. 1976 Mar;307(7960):603–5.

[14] Spaulding S. W., Burrow G. N., Bermudez F., Himmelhoch J. M. The Inhibitory Effect of Lithium on Thyroid Hormone Release in Both Euthyroid and Thyrotoxic Patients. *J Clin Endocrinol Metab*. 1972 Dec;35(6):905–11.

[15] Kendall T., Morriss R., Mayo-Wilson E., Marcus E. Assessment and management of bipolar disorder: summary of updated NICE guidance. *BMJ*. 2014 Sep 25;349(sep25 5):g5673–g5673.

[16] Kessler L., Palla J., Baru J. S., Onyenwenyi C., George A. M., Lucas B. P. Lithium as an Adjunct to Radioactive Iodine for the Treatment of Hyperthyroidism: A Systematic Review and Meta-Analysis. Endocrine Practice. 2014 Jul;20(7):737–45.

[17] Bogazzi F., Bartalena L., Campomori A., Brogioni S., Traino C., de Martino F., Rossi G., Lippi F., Pinchera A., Martino E. Treatment with Lithium Prevents Serum Thyroid Hormone Increase after Thionamide Withdrawal and Radioiodine Therapy in Patients with Graves' Disease. *J Clin Endocrinol Metab*. 2002 Oct;87(10):4490–5.

[18] Mercado M., Mendoza-Zubieta V., Bautista-Osorio R., Espinoza-de los Monteros A. L. Treatment of hyperthyroidism with a combination of methimazole and cholestyramine. *J Clin Endocrinol Metab*. 1996 Sep;81(9):3191–3.

[19] Tsai W. C., Pei D., Wang T. F., Wu D. A., Li J. C., Wei C. L., Lee C. H., Chen S. P., Kuo S. W. The effect of combination therapy with propylthiouracil and cholestyramine in the treatment of Graves' hyperthyroidism. *Clin Endocrinol* (Oxf). 2005 May;62(5):521–4.

[20] Sanders J., Evans M., Betterle C., Sanders P., Bhardwaja A., Young S., Roberts E., Wilmot J., Richards T., Kiddie A., Small K., Platt H., Summerhayes S., Harris R., Reeve M., Coco G., Zanchetta R., Chen S., Furmaniak J., Smith B. R. A Human Monoclonal Autoantibody to the Thyrotropin Receptor with Thyroid-Stimulating Blocking Activity. *Thyroid*. 2008 Jul;18(7):735–46.

[21] Salvi M., Vannucchi G., Beck-Peccoz P. Potential Utility of Rituximab for Graves' Orbitopathy. *J Clin Endocrinol Metab*. 2013 Nov;98(11):4291–9.

[22] Neumann S., Eliseeva E., McCoy J. G., Napolitano G., Giuliani C., Monaco F., Huang W., Gershengorn M. C. A New Small-Molecule Antagonist Inhibits Graves' Disease Antibody Activation of the TSH Receptor. *J Clin Endocrinol Metab*. 2011 Feb 1;96(2):548–54.

Chapter 8

The Role of Nuclear Medicine in the Assessment and Management of Hyperthyroidism

Shelley Simon*
Indirani Muthukrishnan
and Dinesh Kumar Gauthaman
Department of Nuclear Medicine, Apollo Hospitals, Chennai, India

Abstract

Hyperthyroidism is a common benign disorder in nuclear medicine. The clinical diagnosis of hyperthyroidism is confirmed using a primary diagnostic investigation that includes thyroid function tests and ultrasonography. Thyroid scintigraphy remains the investigation of choice to assess the functional status.

Commonly used tests in nuclear medicine are 99mTc-pertechnetate and 2- and 24-hour radioactive iodine uptake. Thyroid scintigraphy distinguishes hyperthyroidism with characteristic patterns of Graves' disease, solitary toxic nodules or toxic multinodular goiter (TMNG), and thyroiditis. Tc-99m sestaMIBI scans were used to differentiate between type I and type II amiodarone-induced thyroiditis and plan for management.

The first line of management for hyperthyroidism is antithyroid drugs, which results in side effects such as allergy, agranulocytosis, and hepatitis on long-term use. Surgery is considered in patients with recurrent Graves' disease, severe ophthalmopathy, or TMNG with

* Corresponding Author's Email: shelleysimon@rediffmail.com.

In: Understanding and Managing Hyperthyroidism
Editor: Poongkodi Karunakaran
ISBN: 979-8-88697-636-6

obstructive symptoms. However, radioiodine treatment for hyperthyroidism is an alternative and effective choice with specific indications and contraindications. It is safe and provides better outcomes. Radiation safety guidelines for the safe use of radionuclides should also be followed.

Keywords: radioiodine, scintigraphy, hyperthyroidism, radioactive iodine

1. Introduction

The thyroid is the first organ to develop in the human embryo; its development begins approximately 22 days after conception. The thyroid gland is the largest endocrine gland in the human body. Adequate levels of thyroid hormones are crucial for the proper functioning of all tissues and organ systems in the body. In an epidemiological study performed in India, subclinical and overt hyperthyroidism were present in 1.6% and 1.3% of the subjects, respectively, who participated in a community survey [1]. This article focuses on the role of nuclear medicine in the assessment and management of patients with hyperthyroidism.

Nuclear thyroidology commenced in the 1930s. Detailed studies of radioiodine physiology led to Hertz and Roberts' first radioactive iodine (RAI) treatment of hyperthyroidism in 1941 [2]. However, the mechanism of sodium iodide symporter (NIS) in iodine uptake in the thyroid gland was described by Kaminsky et al. only in 1993. Nuclear medicine plays a major role in establishing the diagnosis and therapy for thyroid disorders.

1.1. Hyperthyroidism: Definition and Etiology

Hyperthyroidism is a clinical condition characterized by the overproduction of thyroid hormones by the thyroid gland. It can have various causes, of which Graves' disease (GD) and toxic nodular disease are the most common.

In iodine-sufficient populations, autoimmune hyperthyroidism (GD) causes hyperthyroidism, whereas in iodine-deficient populations, toxic multinodular goiter (TMNG), a nonimmune condition, is the most common cause of hyperthyroidism. Approximately 5% of cases are due to toxic thyroid adenomas (TAs); this condition is also called Plummer disease. These thyroid disorders show a female preponderance, with a female-to-male ratio of approximately 6:1. Other rare causes include factitious (exogenous intake) hyperthyroidism and excessive pituitary production of thyroid-stimulating hormone (TSH) due to either a TSH-secreting adenoma or pituitary resistance to thyroid hormones. GD and TA typically occur in the fourth decade of life, whereas TMNG typically occurs between 30 and 60 years of age.

2. Pathophysiology of Hyperthyroidism

Destructive thyroiditis is commonly caused by viral infections and autoimmune thyroid diseases. Thyrotoxicosis results from the destruction of thyroid follicles and release of excessive amounts of preformed thyroid hormones. Thyroiditis is a self-limiting disorder, with the restoration of euthyroidism typically occurring within 3–12 months. Viral thyroiditis is usually associated with painful goiter and does not frequently cause permanent hypothyroidism. Autoimmune thyroiditis is generally associated with painless goiters and increased levels of thyroid peroxidase antibodies. A high incidence of permanent hypothyroidism is observed in the long-term follow-up in patients with destructive thyroiditis. It most commonly occurs in postpartum women due to immune rebound following pregnancy, when the levels of thyroid peroxidase (TPO) antibodies are usually high.

GD is an organ-specific autoimmune disease caused by circulating autoantibodies (generally of the IgG1 isotype) targeting TSH receptors (TSHRs). TSHR autoantibodies (TRAbs) stimulate the thyroid gland after binding to TSH by increasing the production of intracellular cyclic adenosine monophosphate (cAMP). In addition, TRAb interacts with insulin-like growth factor 1 receptors on the surface of thyroid cells and orbital fibroblasts. This activates intracellular cAMP, resulting in thyrocyte hyperplasia, increased vascularity, and increased thyroid hormone production and secretion. TSHR expression is also observed in retroorbital and pretibial tissues, causing extrathyroidal manifestations of the disease. In addition to TRAbs, other antibodies such as antithyroglobulin and antithyroperoxidase antibodies are often present in patients with GD.

Environmental factors, such as dietary iodine, smoking, and emotional stress, can cause the precipitation of GD in genetically predisposed individuals [3, 4]. In addition to genetic susceptibility, smoking acts as a risk factor for GD and Graves' ophthalmopathy. Smoking is associated with GD recurrence, a higher risk of worsening eye changes related to Graves' ophthalmopathy after radioiodine therapy, and a less favorable treatment outcome for Graves' ophthalmopathy with steroids or retrobulbar irradiation.

Table 1. Antibodies in hyperthyroidism

1.	TSH receptor autoantibodies (stimulating)	TRAb
2.	Antithyroglobulin antibodies	Anti-Tg Ab
3.	Anti-thyroperoxidase antibodies	Anti-TPO Ab

In TMNG, nonfunctioning and functioning nodules coexist and, over time, become autonomous, secreting thyroid hormones independently of the circulating levels of TSH, thus causing hyperthyroidism. Nodules in TMNG show a heterogeneous pattern of iodine uptake, displaying either low (cold follicle) or high (hot follicle) iodine uptake on radioiodine scans.

A TA is a benign tumor of monoclonal thyrocytes secreting thyroid hormones in the absence of TSH stimulus in an otherwise normal gland. It results in increased iodine transport and iodination rate and increased expression of thyroperoxidase and sodium iodide symporter mRNA. Iodine deficiency also plays a crucial role in developing thyroid autonomy.

Amiodarone, which is used in patients with paroxysmal and persistent atrial fibrillation, can cause hyperthyroidism. The incidence of amiodarone-induced thyroid dysfunction is up to 24%; hyperthyroidism occurs in 10% of patients. There are two major types of amiodarone-induced thyrotoxicosis (AIT): Type 1 AIT occurs in patients because of excessive iodine-induced hormone synthesis and release, which is called the Jod-Basedow phenomenon, usually seen in patients with preexisting thyroid diseases, such as nodular thyroid glands and endemic goiter regions. Type 2 AIT is destructive thyroiditis, which causes the release of preformed thyroid hormones from damaged thyroid follicular cells, typically seen in patients without underlying thyroid disease.

3. Hyperthyroidism: Clinical Presentation

Overt hyperthyroidism presents with symmetric fine tremor, heat intolerance, sweating, weight loss despite increased appetite, hyperkinesis, nervousness, inability to concentrate, increased metabolic rate, tachycardia, cardiac arrhythmias, hyperdefecation, proximal muscle weakness, oligo- or amenorrhea, emotional instability, and irritability. Young patients usually present with the classic symptoms. In contrast, patients aged >75 years are more likely to present subtle symptoms, such as apathy, fatigue, mood disturbance, and dyspnea. Signs such as atrial fibrillation, congestive heart failure, acute ischemia, and acute coronary syndrome are also more frequent in older people. GD-related thyrotoxicosis occurs in 0.2% of pregnancies.

Infiltrative orbitopathy, dermopathy, and acropachy can occur in patients with GD. Orbitopathy usually presents with irritation of the eyes, injection of the conjunctiva and eyelids, and proptosis, which may lead to lagophthalmos, corneal dryness, ulceration, infection, diplopia, and various degrees of optic neuropathy. Dermopathy occurs less frequently and presents as hyperpigmented, non-pitting edema, generally on the skin of the legs. Decreased bone mineral density occurs in both subclinical and overt hyperthyroidism. However, the less likely causes include hyperthyroidism induced by metastases from well-differentiated thyroid cancers and struma ovarii.

4. Radiopharmaceutical Principles and Instrumentation

4.1. Radiopharmaceuticals

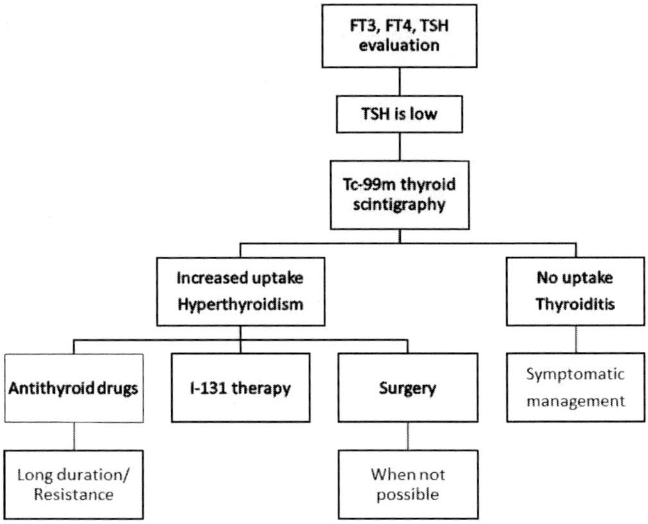

Flow chart representing the role of nuclear medicine in the diagnosis and treatment of hyperthyroidism.

Radiopharmaceuticals used in diagnostic thyroid imaging include radioiodines (I-123, I-131), Technetium 99m (Tc-99m) pertechnetate, and Tc-99m sestaMIBI. Each of these radiopharmaceuticals has its own advantages and disadvantages.

Table 2. Radiotracers for thyroid uptake and imaging

Radiotracer	Administered dose		Route of administration
	In Curies (conventional unit)	**In Becquerels (SI unit)**	
I-123 iodine	200–400 μCi#	7.4–14.8 MBq$	oral
I-131 iodine	5 μCi	0.19 MBq	oral
Tc-99m pertechnetate	5–10 mCi£	185–370 MBq	i.v.¥
Tc-99m sestaMIBI	5–10 mCi	185–370 MBq	i.v.

*I-131 radioiodine is used only for uptake measurement and not for diagnostic imaging, because higher activity needed for imaging is associated with a high absorbed radiation dose to the thyroid gland.

#μCi – microcurie

$MBq – megabecquerel

£ mCi – millicurie

¥i.v. - intravenous

4.1.1. Technetium-99m

Tc-99m is intravenously administered in the form of 99mTcO4- Na (sodium pertechnetate) eluted from a molybdenum-technetium generator. The advantages of Tc-99m are its high availability, low energy of gamma photons (140 keV), and a shorter half-life (6 hours). These characteristics allow for obtaining more accurate images in a shorter scan acquisition time and with an absorbed dose much lower than that with diagnostic I-131 activity. Tc-99m is biomimetic, that is, it is transported into thyrocytes, similar to iodine isotopes, by the NIS. However, it does not undergo organification, as in the case of iodine isotopes. Maximal accumulation of Tc-99m-pertechnetate is achieved 15–20 min after its intravenous administration [5, 6].

4.1.1.1. Measurement of Technetium-99m Uptake (Using a Gamma Camera)

In a euthyroid and iodine-sufficient population, the maximum uptake of Tc-99m is 0.5–2.0% of the administered activity. Similar to iodine uptake, the Tc-99m uptake percentage is lower in hypothyroidism, iodine contamination, and subacute thyroiditis and higher in GD and iodine deficiency. This measurement technique is simple and performed as a supplement to thyroid scintigraphy by comparing the number of counts in the thyroid with the number of counts in the syringe containing the Tc-99m-pertechnetate prior to injection (both corrected by background subtraction); more precise information is provided by uptake probes [5, 6].

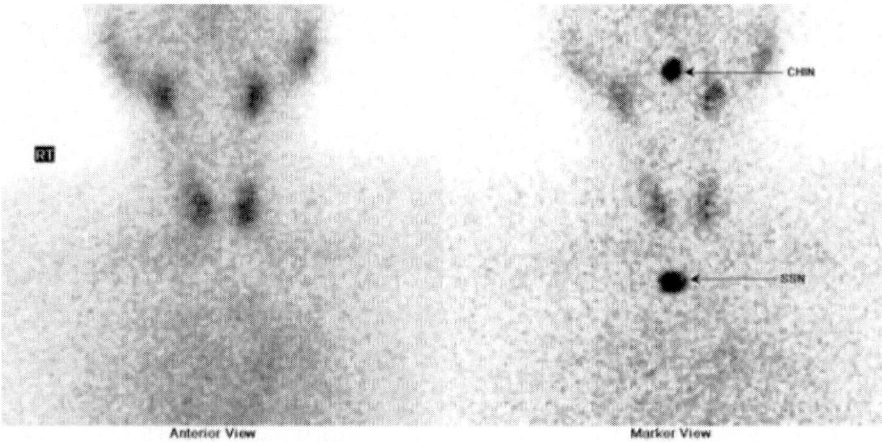

Figure 1. Technetium-99m thyroid scintigraphy (planar two-dimensional imaging): Normal scan showing homogenous tracer (technetium-99m) uptake in both lobes of the thyroid gland and physiological tracer uptake in the bilateral parotid and submandibular glands.

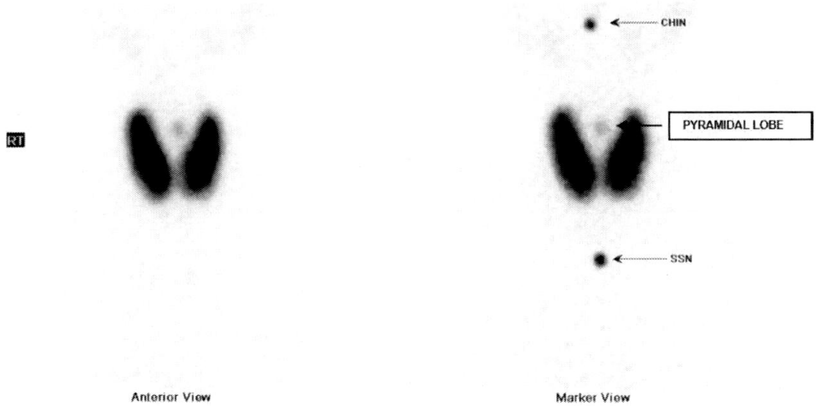

Figure 2. Technetium-99m thyroid scintigraphy: Graves' disease showing diffuse homogenously increased tracer uptake in both lobes of the thyroid gland, which are enlarged, and suppression of the physiological tracer uptake in the bilateral salivary glands. Faint visualization of the pyramidal lobe is noted.

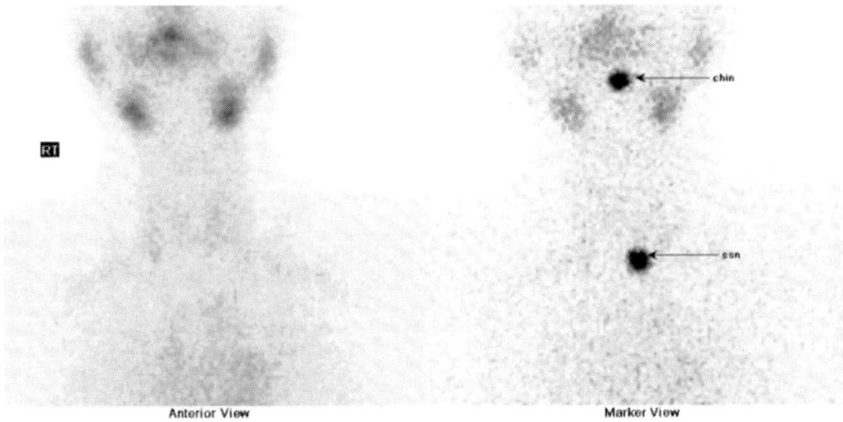

Figure 3. Technetium-99m thyroid scintigraphy: Subacute thyroiditis showing poor or no tracer uptake by the thyroid gland and physiological tracer uptake in the bilateral salivary glands.

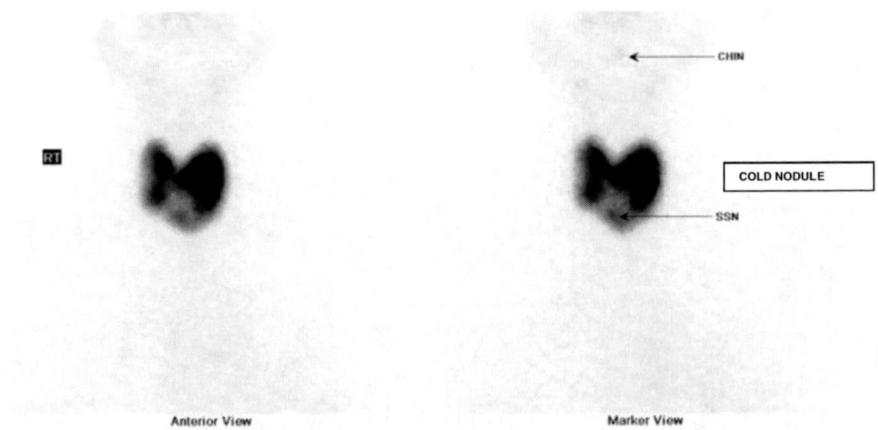

Figure 4. Technetium-99m thyroid scintigraphy: Toxic multinodular goiter showing heterogeneously increased tracer uptake in both lobes of the enlarged thyroid gland, with few cold areas (areas of reduced tracer uptake), and suppressed physiological tracer uptake in the bilateral salivary glands. Fine needle aspiration cytology must be performed to rule out malignancy in the cold nodules before planning for I-131 therapy.

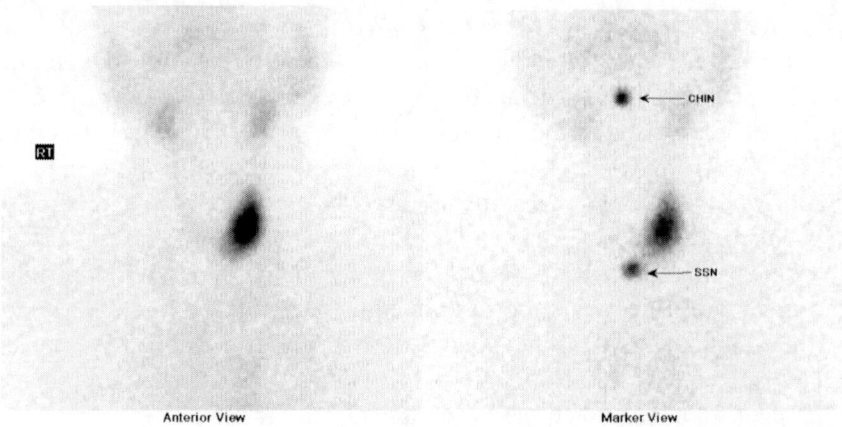

Figure 5. Technetium-99m thyroid scintigraphy: Toxic adenoma showing focal increased tracer uptake in the left lobe of the thyroid gland (corresponding to clinically palpable nodule) with suppression of tracer uptake in the rest of the thyroid parenchyma in both lobes and physiological tracer uptake in the bilateral salivary glands.

4.1.2. Iodine isotopes: I-123 and I-131

I-123 is a pure gamma emitter with a low energy (159 keV) and short half-life (13 hours) of gamma photons. The advantage of I-123 is its higher specificity and persistent accumulation in the thyroid due to organification, which allows delayed acquisition and detailed assessment of iodine kinetics in the thyroid. Compared with Tc-99m, I-123 images have better thyroid resolution and visualization of the retrosternal thyroid and thyroid gland when the thyroid uptake is low. Iodine turnover in the thyroid can be assessed with I-123, whereas Tc-99m uptake is only a surrogate parameter. However, the low availability and high cost of I-123 make its routine use difficult.

I-131, the most commonly used radioactive isotope of iodine, emits beta and gamma radiation with a half-life of 8.1 days. Its gamma rays are used for diagnostic purposes, which have a higher energy of 364 keV than I-123, and its beta energy is used for therapeutic purposes (beta max: 606 keV). Therefore, I-131 scintigraphy should be limited to dosimetric pretreatment evaluations of patients with thyrotoxicosis and well-differentiated thyroid cancers, as well as in the follow-up of patients with differentiated thyroid cancer, ectopic thyroid imaging (i.e., retrosternal or lingual thyroid, and struma ovarii), and kinetic studies in dyshormonogenetic pathologies [5-8].

4.1.2.1. Measurement of Radioiodine Uptake

RAI uptake test (RAIU) is performed using a gamma probe positioned at a distance from the patient's neck. Uptake measurements were performed at various time intervals after the oral administration of 100 microcurie (μCi) of I-123 or 50 μCi of I-131. I-131 is commonly used because of its limited availability of I-123. A gamma camera is used for imaging and uptake studies. Measurements taken in the first 24 hours are essential for the assessment of iodine kinetics in the thyroid gland. Hence, depending on the requirements, iodine uptake measurements are performed at standard 2, 24, and 48 hours after the administration of the diagnostic dose of radioiodine. Whenever imaging is planned, 100–150 μCi of I-131 is administered, and uptake measurements are performed before the scheduled radioiodine imaging. It is commonly higher in hyperthyroidism and lower in hypothyroidism, and the values need to be standardized for the nuclear medicine department. Many factors (mostly iatrogenic) other than the thyroid functional status may influence the level of thyroid iodine uptake [5]. In the pediatric population, the dose administered is adjusted to the patient's weight (Young's formula: $\frac{\text{Age in years}}{\text{Age+12}}$ x adult dose).

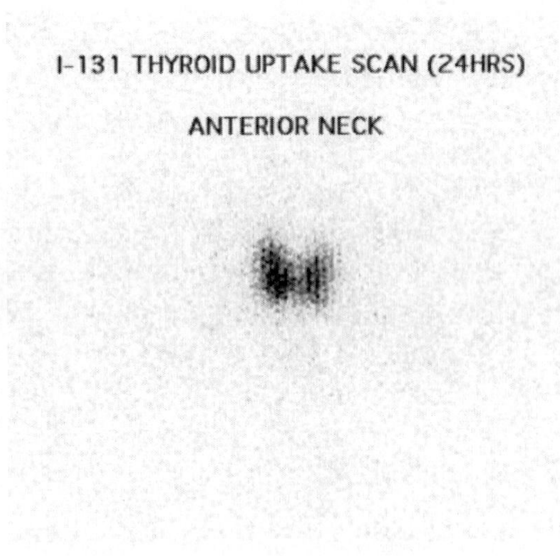

Figure 6. I-131 thyroid scintigraphy (planar two-dimensional imaging): Normal scan showing homogenous tracer (I-131) uptake in both lobes of the thyroid gland. The physiological tracer uptake in the bilateral parotid and submandibular glands is faintly visualized because of the low image resolution of I-131 scintigraphy compared with technetium-99m thyroid scintigraphy.

Figure 7. I-131 thyroid scintigraphy: Graves' disease showing diffuse homogenously increased tracer uptake in both lobes of the thyroid gland.

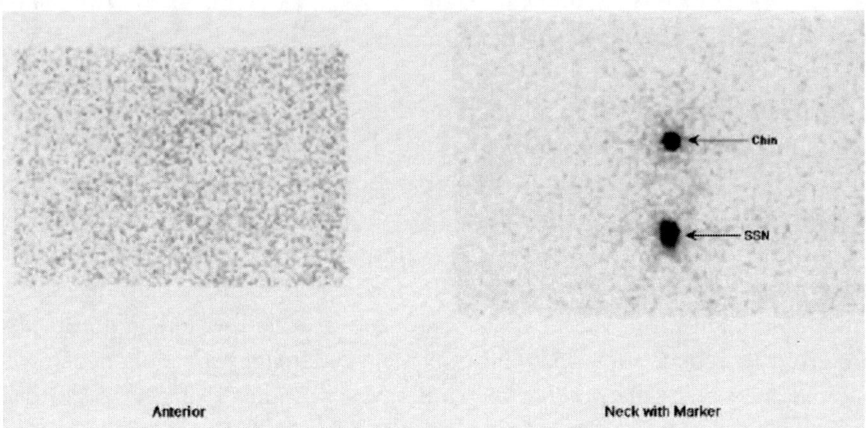

Figure 8. I-131 thyroid scintigraphy: Subacute thyroiditis showing poor or no tracer uptake by the thyroid gland

4.2. Instrumentation

Following radiotracer administration, the patient becomes a source of radiation. Several devices are used to detect and capture these emissions (gamma, beta-negative, beta-positive) and convert them into photons, parametric images, numbers, and molecular information, as follows:

1. Rectilinear scanner, which is the oldest imaging device, is no longer being used.
2. Gamma camera planar scanner, which is the most widely used nuclear medicine device for the diagnosis of benign thyroid diseases, provides segmental two-dimensional (2D) images, whole body reconstructions, and dynamic acquisitions.
3. A single-photon emission computed tomography (SPECT) scanner, which is a 3D tomographic device that uses gamma camera data from various projections reconstructed in different planes, can be fused with computed tomography (CT).
4. Positron emission tomography (PET)-CT scanner, which is CT-aided PET.

4.3. Thyroid Scintigraphy

4.3.1. Patient Preparation, Instrumentation, and Image Acquisition

Thyroid scintigraphy is performed using a gamma camera with SPECT or SPECT/CT. No prior strict patient preparation is needed for Tc-99m thyroid scintigraphy. It is not necessary to follow any special diet or suspend the usual medications. However, when I-131 scintigraphy is being planned, it is mandatory for patients to discontinue medicines such as carbimazole or propylthiouracil for at least 7 days before the scan. A low-iodine diet is also preferred to reduce dietary iodine interference. Images are obtained in the anterior view with the pinhole or parallelhole collimator placed as close as possible to the patient's extended neck. The duration of the image is approximately 5 min. SPECT/CT is performed to study the thyroid nodules, ectopic thyroid glands, and intrathoracic goiters.

4.3.2. Scan Interpretation

Normal thyroid scintigraphy shows the thyroid gland with symmetrical lobes, and the lateral borders of the lobes are straight-to-convex with homogenous tracer distribution. Radiotracers are also normally observed in the salivary glands, vessels, and soft tissues.

Hyperfunctioning thyroid tissue shows markedly increased uptake of radioiodine (I-123 or I-131) or Tc-99m pertechnetate. The patterns of scan findings determine the different forms of hyperthyroidism. In GD, the tracer distribution is homogenous, primarily because this hyperfunction results from circulating TRAbs, which target all TSHR-expressing thyroid cells, thus occasionally resulting in the visualization of the pyramidal lobe.

In TA, increased tracer uptake is confined to hyperfunctioning nodule/nodules. The normal thyroid parenchyma outside the nodule is in a dormant state and, therefore, does not or shows a very low concentration of radioiodine or Tc-99m pertechnetate because TSH secretion is suppressed in a hyperthyroid state. In TMNG, heterogeneous nodular uptake is noted in different nodules. Regions without uptake are also noted within large hyperfunctioning nodules, reflecting areas of regression. In GD and TMNG, physiological tracer uptake in the salivary glands is often markedly reduced or absent.

Based on the concentration of tracer uptake, functioning thyroid nodules can be hot or warm (increased uptake) and nonfunctioning nodules are cold (no uptake). This assessment of uptake is vital for the stratification of malignancy risk. The highest probability of malignancy is found in cold nodules.

The diagnosis of GD does not exclude the presence of thyroid nodules. Hyperthyroidism of autoimmune origin with coexisting nodular focal lesions in the thyroid is known as Marine-Lenhart syndrome. Thyroid scintigraphy in this condition is of significant value since the risk of thyroid cancer in a cold nodule in GD is higher than that in a cold nodule without autoimmune thyroid disease, estimated at 15–19%. In addition, thyroid cancer coexisting with GD is clinically more aggressive, which could be explained by the stimulating effect of thyroid antibodies [9].

Thyroid scintigraphy shows marked heterogeneity due to reduced or absent tracer uptake in the hyperthyroid phase of thyroiditis. Poor-to-patchy heterogeneous tracer uptake is noted in the recovery phase of thyroiditis. Low or absent uptake is observed in thyrotoxicosis factitia due to the suppressive effects of exogenous T4.

In AIT, both type 1 and 2 AIT patients show reduced or no visualization of the gland on thyroid scintigraphy. Type 1 AIT cannot be distinguished from type 2 AIT using radioiodine or Tc-99m pertechnetate thyroid scintigraphy. However, the two types of AIT can be distinguished using a different tracer called Tc-99m sestaMIBI, which shows preserved tracer uptake in type 1 and reduced or absent tracer uptake in type 2 AIT [10].

False positive tracer uptake is noted in situations such as

- Functional NIS expression in normal tissues, including the thymus, breast, salivary glands, gastrointestinal tract, and various benign and malignant tumors
- Metabolism of radioiodinated thyroid hormones
- Retention or contamination by radioiodinated body fluids (e.g., saliva, tears, blood, urine, exudate, transudate, gastric, and mucosal secretions)
- Retention and uptake of radioiodine in inflamed tissues
- Thyroid metastasis

5. Treatment Options for Hyperthyroidism

The therapeutic options available for treating hyperthyroidism include antithyroid drugs, surgery, and radioiodine therapy (I-131). The primary line of initial management is the antithyroid drugs propylthiouracil and carbimazole, which act at different steps of iodination, such as iodine concentration, iodine organification, and synthesis or release of thyroid hormones. Surgery includes thyroidectomy. The disease recurrence rate after tapering the dose or cessation of therapy is high, constituting >90% in TMNG and 40–50% in GD. Antithyroid drug treatment must be continued for months to years to minimize the disease recurrence rates. However, patients being treated with long-term medical therapy may develop adverse reactions, ranging from minor (skin rashes) to major (e.g., agranulocytosis or hepatitis). Therefore, these patients must undergo regular laboratory studies and clinical follow-up visits.

Surgery is usually reserved for selected patients with recurrent GD or TMNG uncontrolled by medical therapy and in the abnormally enlarged thyroid gland that causes a mass effect, compressing neighboring structures. Surgery is also indicated in patients with severe Graves' ophthalmopathy with contraindications to I-131 therapy or failed response to radioiodine therapy.

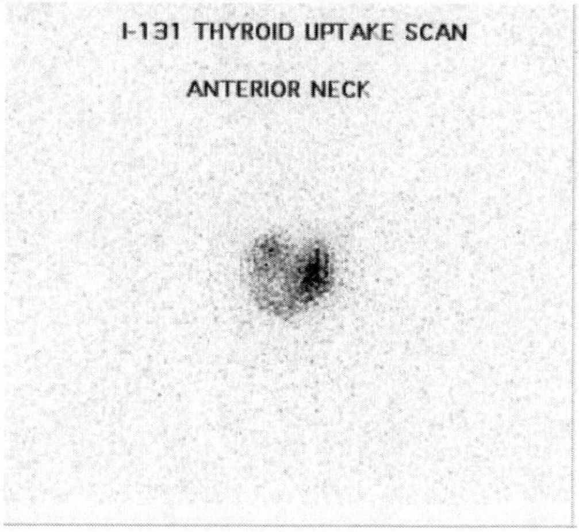

Figure 9. I-131 thyroid scintigraphy: Toxic multinodular goiter showing heterogeneously increased tracer uptake in both lobes of the enlarged thyroid gland, with cold areas (areas of reduced tracer uptake) in the right lobe.

I-131 is an effective method for treating hyperthyroidism, which induces apoptosis or necrobiosis of most of the hyperfunctioning cells but not all thyroid cells. Thus, sufficient viable thyroid parenchyma is left behind to ensure the production of thyroid hormones and maintain their circulating levels within normal values.

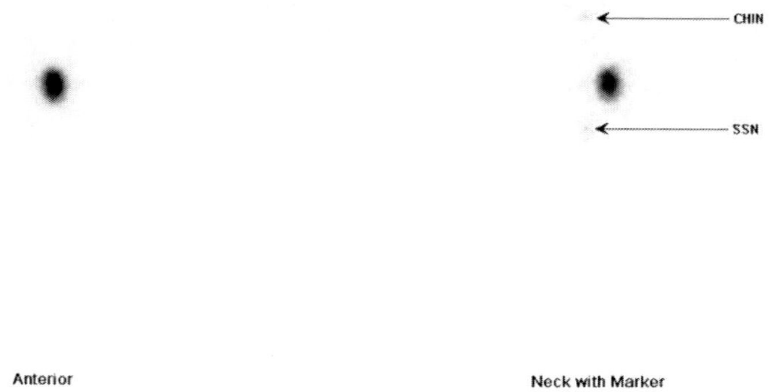

Figure 10. I-131 thyroid scintigraphy: Toxic adenoma showing increased focal tracer uptake in the left lobe of the thyroid gland (corresponding to clinically palpable nodule) and suppressed tracer uptake in the rest of the thyroid parenchyma in both lobes.

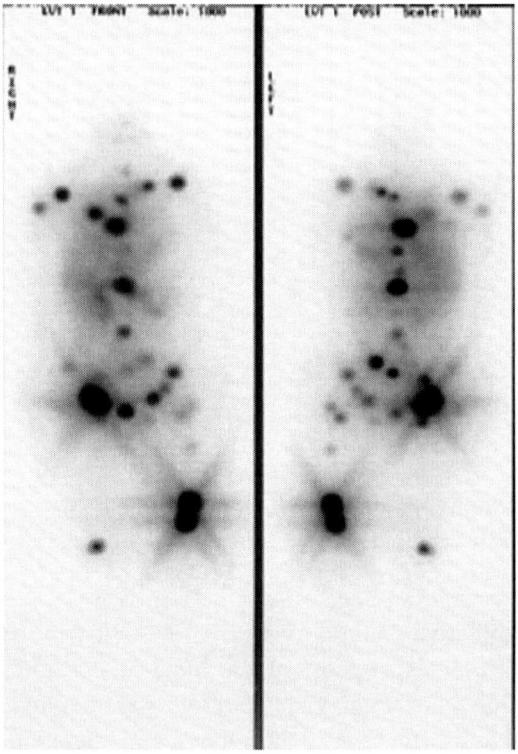

Figure 11. Whole body I-131 scintigraphy in a known metastatic differentiated thyroid carcinoma patient, post thyroidectomy, showing multiple foci of I-131 avid skeletal metastases – functional thyroid metastases resulting in hyperthyroidism.

5.1. Mechanism of Action of Radioactive Iodine I-131

Beta particles emitted by I-131 are responsible for the majority of radiobiological effects of this radioisotope. The maximum energy of these beta particles is 0.61 MeV, and the average range in soft tissues is approximately 0.4 mm, with a maximum range of approximately 3 mm. The radiobiological effects of I-131 in tissues could be direct single- or double-strand DNA damage resulting in radiation-induced apoptosis or necrobiosis (cell death) or indirect damage caused by free radicals produced by the interaction of radiation with water, which interacts with critical macromolecules in the cell. This combined radiobiologic effect induces cellular apoptosis and destruction of the thyroid follicles, replacing them with fibrotic tissue. Therefore, the ultimate effect of radioiodine therapy is comparable to that of surgical removal of the thyroid tissue.

In GD, I-131 therapy produces a hypothyroid status. Here, all thyroid cells are exposed to stimulation with circulating TRAbs. Even if a euthyroid status is achieved after radioiodine therapy, it is short-lived because of persistent circulating TRAbs. The residual viable thyroid cells undergo continuous stimulation, and sooner or later, the disease recurs. To prevent this, the goal of radioiodine therapy is to render the patients permanently hypothyroid, a condition that can be treated with oral thyroid hormone replacement therapy [11, 12].

In contrast, in TMNG or TA, the euthyroid state is achievable because only nodules bearing the somatic mutation cause autonomous activation of the TSHR and concentrate radioiodine. The extranodular thyroid spares radiobiological damage. When the hyperfunctioning nodules regress, the extranodular parenchyma resumes functioning.

5.2. Indications and Contraindications

The American Thyroid Association guidelines of 2016 [11] list the following clinical conditions that indicate radioiodine therapy, in addition to intolerance or resistance to antithyroid drugs: comorbidities that increase the general surgical risk; prior neck surgery or irradiation of the neck; lack of access to a high-volume thyroid surgeon; and periodic thyrotoxic hypokalemic paralysis, right heart failure due to pulmonary hypertension, or congestive heart failure. In addition to the indications mentioned above, the 2018 European Thyroid Association guideline for the management of Graves hyperthyroidism [12] recommends considering radioiodine therapy also in cases of mild hyperthyroidism (even with a serum TSH level of between 0.1 and 0.39 mIU/mL), given the high potential for progression of this condition to a more severe state of hyperthyroidism and increased risk of acute cardiac events and mortality—especially in patients aged >65 years.

I-131 radioiodine therapy for hyperthyroidism is an absolute contraindication to pregnant and lactating women. Other contraindications (considered absolute by some guidelines and relative by other guidelines) include the inability to adhere to radiation safety recommendations, coexisting or suspected thyroid cancer, pregnancy planned within 6 months of radioiodine therapy, and uncontrolled hyperthyroidism. Radioiodine therapy should be considered with great caution in patients with Graves' ophthalmopathy (especially smokers) because cell damage induced by radiation results in the release of thyroid antigens into the circulation, which enhances immunogenic stimulation leading to TRAb production, thereby promoting de novo or worsening Graves' orbitopathy [13, 14].

5.3. Radioiodine Therapy

A detailed clinical history is essential to administer radioiodine therapy. The patient must provide a thorough medical history regarding previous treatments with antithyroid drugs, radiographic studies with iodinated contrast medium, therapy with amiodarone or other iodine-containing medications, and recent consumption of iodine-rich food or procedures.

Complete patient workup, including laboratory tests to confirm hyperthyroidism, thyroid scintigraphy, RAIU and scanning, ultrasonography to assess the thyroid target volume (or MRI in cases of intrathoracic extension), and a negative pregnancy test in women of childbearing age need to be performed [15]. Fine needle aspiration of thyroid nodules, especially those that appear hypofunctioning on thyroid scintigraphy (i.e., cold nodules), should be performed to rule out malignancy. In patients with large goiters (especially those >80 cm3 with intrathoracic extension), radiation-induced inflammation may result in swelling of the thyroid parenchyma, causing narrowing of the tracheal lumen, especially in long-standing bulky goiters, which weakens the cartilage structure of the trachea. The physician must explain the procedure, possible complications and side effects, therapeutic alternatives, and expected outcomes in detail and obtain informed consent from the patients. Lactating mothers must be advised to stop breastfeeding, and therapy should be delayed until lactation ceases, so as to minimize the radiation dose to both the child and the breast.

5.3.1. Patient Preparation

Preparation for radioiodine therapy is aimed at optimizing the concentration of I-131 radioiodine in the hyperfunctioning thyroid parenchyma (the whole gland in GD, hyperfunctioning nodules in TMNG, and TA). Antithyroid drugs must be discontinued for at least 2–3 weeks in case of carbimazole and methimazole and at least 3 days in case of propylthiouracil. If the symptoms of hyperthyroidism recur during the interval of drug withdrawal, beta-blockers can be used to control the symptoms. In hyperthyroid patients for whom radioiodine therapy is selected as the first-line treatment, a brief course of antithyroid drug treatment is suggested to deplete the intrathyroidal hormone stores by blocking iodination of tyrosine residues while the gland continues to respond to TRAbs by releasing previously formed thyroid hormone, especially in elderly patients and patients with preexisting heart disease or severe systemic illness [15]. Patients must discontinue the use of iodine-containing medications for at least 2–3 weeks, except amiodarone, which requires withdrawal for months with monitoring of urinary iodine excretion [16]. Although many European centers prepare patients with a low-iodine diet for 10–15 days before administering radioiodine therapy, in the United States, the low-iodine diet is reserved for patients with thyroid cancer. Some centers prescribe lithium 7 days before administering radioiodine (250 mg three times daily) to block radioiodine release from the thyroid gland without interfering with its uptake [17]; however, this practice has not been widely used.

5.3.2. Dosimetry

The dose of I-131 to treat hyperthyroidism remains a matter of debate. A practical approach is to administer a fixed empirical activity (185, 370, or 555 megabecquerel [MBq], that is, 5, 10, and 15 millicurie [mCi], respectively) based on the severity and duration of thyrotoxicosis, size of the goiter, RAIU value, and past medications [18]. Therapy is administered as an outpatient or inpatient procedure according to the radiation regulatory requirements of the country. Alternatively, the I-131 radioiodine activity for hyperthyroidism therapy is based on applying a fixed value of the target absorbed dose on medical internal radiation dose formulations using the thyroid gland size and 24-hour RAIU value (38) or the effective radioiodine half-life in the thyroid gland. Recommended radiation doses range from 150 to 300 Gray (Gy) for GD and from 300 to 400 Gy for autonomously functioning nodules [19]. Multinodular goiters usually require the administration of relatively high doses of I-131 radioiodine because the thyroid is large and RAI distribution is heterogeneous. To maximize the gastrointestinal absorption rate of orally administered I-131 radioiodine, patients are required to fast for at least 4 hours before therapy and drink at least 1 L of water in the hour after treatment.

5.3.3. Effectiveness of Therapy and Patient Follow Up

Fixed-dose I-131 radioiodine therapy is very successful in 80% of patients. Euthyroidism is usually achieved within 3–12 months after therapy. Patients who fail to respond can undergo a second treatment, which is effective in approximately 90% of the cases. A second dose of I-131 therapy is needed, especially in patients with long-standing thyrotoxicosis, longer duration of medical management, and problems with intestinal absorption such as malabsorption syndrome. Surgery should be considered in patients who do not respond even after the two doses of radioiodine therapy.

The effectiveness of radioiodine therapy for hyperthyroidism is evaluated using clinical and laboratory parameters, usually at 3, 6, and 12 months after treatment [11]. Patients with GD should be evaluated for either euthyroidism or hypothyroidism. Long-term follow-up is recommended, so that L-thyroxine supplementation can be initiated. For patients with hyperfunctioning thyroid nodules, the treatment goal is to achieve euthyroidism, as well as to reduce volume, which may be assessed using ultrasound and, occasionally, thyroid scintigraphy.

5.3.4. Delayed Side Effects

It is crucial to follow-up patients undergoing radioiodine therapy as hypothyroidism develops at a rate of approximately 5% per year after the therapy. Hypothyroidism occurs in <10% of patients with a solitary toxic nodule who are administered radioiodine therapy. In patients with TMNG, the incidence of hypothyroidism ranges between 20% and 75% within 8 years after radioiodine therapy [20].

Ophthalmopathy may occur or worsen if already present in patients with GD after radioiodine therapy, particularly in smokers, patients with severe hyperthyroidism and high TRAb levels, and patients with a recent onset of hyperthyroidism. This effect is due to the release of thyroid antigens by damaged thyroid cells, resulting in the stimulation of immune events associated with ophthalmopathy [13, 14]. When radioiodine therapy is planned for patients with ophthalmopathy, oral corticosteroid prophylaxis may be considered to minimize the exacerbation of ophthalmopathy. However, its usefulness has not yet been proven. Although reduced fertility is a common concern, it is unlikely to occur with a relatively low dose treatment administered to patients with hyperthyroidism. However, there are few recommendations for conception after therapy, at least 6 months in women and 4 months in men, to allow turnover of ovum and spermatogenesis, as well as to ensure that the patient is euthyroid and on a stable dose of hormone replacement. The widespread fear of radiation-induced malignancies after radioiodine therapy in patients with thyroid cancers is not new, although it is not justified by follow-up data. A similar concern has been raised for hyperthyroidism, which has been strongly refuted [21, 22, 23, 24].

6. Neonatal Hyperthyroidism

Hyperthyroidism in newborns is caused by the passage of maternal TRAbs into fetal circulation; this may occur if the mother is inadequately treated with propylthiouracil or methimazole, which reduces the levels of these antibodies in GD. As this condition is clinically diagnosed, nuclear medicine has no significant role in it.

Conclusion

The nuclear medicine diagnostic tests for hyperthyroidism are cost-effective, simple, and readily available, and radioiodine I-131 therapy is noninvasive, cost-effective, and has fewer side effects. Patients treated with I-131 need to be followed up with thyroid function tests to decide on the initiation of thyroxine replacement therapy or administration of a second dose of I-131 therapy, whichever is required. The fear of radiation should be overcome, as the literature review states, and I-131 therapy can be administered to the young and reproductive age groups when warranted, according to the guidelines. In conclusion, nuclear medicine plays a crucial role in the assessment and treatment of hyperthyroidism.

References

[1] Usha Menon, V., Sundaram, K. R., Unnikrishnan, A. G., Jayakumar, R. V., Nair, V., and Kumar, H. (2009). High prevalence of undetected thyroid disorders in an iodine sufficient adult south Indian population. *J Indian Med Assoc.*, 107, 72–7.

[2] Sawin, C. T., Becker, D. V. (1997). Radioiodine and the treatment of hyperthyroidism: the early history. *Thyroid*, 7, 163-176.

[3] Laurberg, P., Pedersen, K. M., Vestergaard, H., and Sigurdsson, G. (1991). High incidence of multinodular toxic goitre in the elderly population in a low iodine intake area vs. high incidence of Graves' disease in the young in a high iodine intake area: comparative surveys of thyrotoxicosis epidemiology in East-Jutland Denmark and Iceland. *J Intern Med.*, 229, 415–420.

[4] Eschler, D. C., Hasham, A., and Tomer, Y. (2011). Cutting edge: the etiology of autoimmune thyroid diseases. *Clin Rev Allergy Immunol.*, 41, 190–197.

[5] Czepczynski, R. (2012). Nuclear medicine in the diagnosis of benign thyroid diseases. *Nuclear Med Rev.*, 15. 113–119.

[6] Meller, J., and Becker, W. (2002). The continuing importance of thyroid scintigraphy in the era of high-resolution ultrasound. *Eur J Nucl Med*, 29(suppl 2), S425–S438.

[7] Gharib, H., Papini, E., Paschke, R., Duick, D., Valcavi, R., Hegedüs, L., and Vitti, P. (2010). American Association of Clinical Endocrinologists, Associazione Medici Endocrinologi and European Thyroid Association medical guidelines for clinical practice for the diagnosis and management of thyroid nodules. *EndocrPract*, 16(suppl 1), 1–43.

[8] American Thyroid Association (ATA) Guidelines Taskforce on Thyroid Nodules and Differentiated Thyroid Cancer. Cooper, D. S., Doherty, G. M., Haugen, B. R., Kloos, R. T., Lee, S. L., Mandel, S. J., Mazzaferri, E. L., McIver, B., Pacini, F., Schlumberger, M., Sherman, S. I., Steward, D. L., and Tuttle, R. M. (2009). Revised American Thyroid Association management guidelines for patients with thyroid nodules and differentiated thyroid cancer. *Thyroid*, 19. 1167–1214.

[9] Carnell, N. E., and Valente, W. A. (1998). Thyroid nodules in Graves' disease: classifica-tion, characterization, and response to treatment. *Thyroid*, 8. 1079.

[10] Piga, M., Cocco, M. C., Serra, A., Boi, F., Loy, M., and Mariotti, S. (2008). The usefulness of 99mTc-sestaMIBI thyroid scan in the differential diagnosis and management of amiodarone- induced thyrotoxicosis. *Eur J Endocrinol.*, 159. 423–429.

[11] Ross, D. S., Burch, H. B., Cooper, D. S., Greenlee, M. C., Laurberg, P., Maia, A. L., Rivkees S. A., Samuels, M., Sosa, J. A., Stan, M. N., and Walter, M. A. (2016) American Thyroid Association guidelines for diagnosis and management of hyperthyroidism and other causes of thyrotoxicosis. *Thyroid.*, 26. 1343–1421.

[12] Kahaly, G. J., Bartalena, L., Heged¨us, L., Leenhardt, L., Poppe, K., and Pearce, S. H. (2018). European Thyroid Association guideline for the management of Graves' hyperthyroidism. *Eur Thyroid J.*, 7. 167–186.

[13] Acharya, S. H., Avenell, A., Philip, S., Burr, J., Bevan, J. S., and Abraham, P. (2008). Radioiodine therapy (RAI) for Graves' disease (GD) and the effect on ophthalmopathy: a systematic review. *Clin Endocrinol (Oxf)*. 69. 943–950.

[14] Laurberg, P., Wallin, G., Tallstedt, L., Abraham-Nordling, M., Lundell, G., and Torring, O. (2008). TSH-receptor autoimmunity in Graves' disease after therapy with anti-thyroid drugs, surgery, or radioiodine: a 5-year prospective randomized study. *Eur J Endocrinol.*, 158. 69–75.

[15] Stokkel, M. P. M., Handkiewicz Junak, D., Lassmann, M., Dietlin, M., and Luster, M. (2010). EANM procedure guidelines for therapy of benign thyroid disease. *Eur J Nucl Med Mol Imaging.*, 37. 2218–2228.

[16] Silberstein, E. B., Alavi, A., Balon, H. R., Clarke, S. E., Divgi, C., Gelfand, M. J., Goldsmith S. J., Jadvar, H., Marcus, C. S., Martin, W. H., Parker, J. A., Royal, H. D., Sarkar, S. D., Stabin, M., and Waxman, A. D. (2012). The SNMMI practice guideline for therapy of thyroid disease with 131I 3.0. *J Nucl Med.*, 53. 1633–1651.

[17] Bal, C. S., Kumar, A., and Pandey, R. M. (2002). A randomized controlled trial to evaluate the adjuvant effect of lithium on radioiodine treatment of hyperthyroidism. *Thyroid.*, 12. 399–405.

[18] Marinelli, L. D., Quimby, E. H., and Hine, G. J. (1948). Dosage determination with radioactive isotopes; practical considerations in therapy and protection. *Am J Roentgenol Radium Ther.*, 59. 260–281.

[19] Hänscheid, H., Canzi, C., Eschner, W., Flux, G., Luster, M., Strigari, L., and Lassmann, M. (2013). EANM Dosimetry Committee series on standard operational procedures for pre-therapeutic dosimetry II. Dosimetry prior to radioiodine therapy of benign thyroid diseases. *Eur J Nucl Med Mol Imaging.*, 40, 1126–1134.

[20] Kahraman, D., Keller, C., Schneider, C., Eschner, W., Sudbrock, F., Schmidt, M., Schicha, H., Dietlein, M., and Kobe, C. (2012). Development of hypothyroidism during long-term follow-up of patients with toxic nodular goitre after radioiodine therapy. *Clin Endocrinol (Oxf).*, 76, 297–303.

[21] Subramanian, S., Goldstein, D. P., Parlea, L., Thabane, L, Ezzat, S., Ibrahim-Zada, I., Straus, S., Brierley, J. D., Tsang, R. W., Gafni, A., Rotstein, L., and Sawka, A. M. (2007). Second primary malignancy risk in thyroid cancer survivors: a systematic review and meta-analysis. *Thyroid.*, 17, 1277–1288.

[22] Kitahara, C., Berrington de Gonzalez, A., Bouville, A., Brill, A., Doody, M., Melo D., Simon, S., Sosa, J., Tulchinsky, M., Villoing, D., and Preston, D. (2019). Association of radioactive iodine treatment with cancer mortality in patients with hyperthyroidism. *JAMA Intern Med.*, 179, 1034–1042.

[23] Taylor, P. N., Okosieme, E. O., Chatterjee, K., and Boelaert, K. (2020). Joint statement from the Society for Endocrinology and the British Thyroid Association regarding "association of radioactive iodine treatment with cancer mortality in patients with hyperthyroidism." *Clin Endocrinol (Oxf).*, 92, 266–267.

[24] Giovanella, L., Verburg, F., Ovčariček, P., Iakovou, I., Mihailovic, J., Vrachimis, A, Zerdoud, S., Hoffmann, M., and Luster, M. (2020). "Quid autem vides festucam in oculo fratris tui et trabem in oculo tuo non vide" on the hyperthyroidism-induced mortality and antithyroid drug-induced side effects in the era of radioiodine fake news. European *Journal of Nuclear Medicine and Molecular Imaging.*, 47(6), 1342-1344.

Chapter 9

The Surgical Management of Graves' Disease

Ramakanth Bhargav Panchangam[1,*]
Sabaretnam Mayilvaganan[2,†]
Anand Kumar Mishra[3,‡]
and Poongkodi Karunakaran[4,5,6§]
[1]BGH, Vijayawada, AP, India
[2]SGPGIMS, Lucknow, India
[3]King George's Medical University, Lucknow, India
[4]Endocrine Surgery Unit, Government Mohan Kumaramangalam Medical College, Salem, India
[5]Department of Endocrine Surgery, Madras Medical College, Chennai, India
[6]The Tamilnadu Dr. MGR Medical University, Chennai, India

Abstract

Graves' disease is the most common cause of hyperthyroidism. Antithyroid therapy is the initial modality of treatment which is associated with remission in up to 35% of cases. Definitive therapeutic options after the failure of medical therapy include radioactive iodine ablation and surgical removal of the gland. Both these modalities need life-long thyroxine replacement. In recent years, there is increasing interest in the surgical management of Graves' disease. Total thyroidectomy or near total thyroidectomy is considered the procedure of choice as it offers an immediate and permanent cure for hyperthyroidism and incidental thyroid cancers. However, total thyroidectomy is

* Corresponding Author's Email: endoanswers@gmail.com.
† Corresponding Author's Email: drretnam@gmail.com.
‡ Corresponding Author's Email: poongkodithesurgeon@gmail.com.
§ Corresponding Author's Email: mishra101@gmail.com.

In: Understanding and Managing Hyperthyroidism
Editor: Poongkodi Karunakaran
ISBN: 979-8-88697-636-6

associated with higher rates of postoperative hypoparathyroidism and laryngeal nerve injuries compared to lesser resective surgery. This chapter deals with the indications for surgery in Graves' disease, surgical techniques, and its complications. It also deals with innovative technology, the role of endoscopic thyroidectomy, and surgical adjuncts available to improve the safety and efficacy of surgery.

Keywords: thyroidectomy, open total thyroidectomy, endoscopic thyroidectomy, surgery

1. Introduction

Graves' disease (GD) is one of the most common endocrine diseases. GD is also the most common cause of thyrotoxicosis. The differential diagnosis includes many other types of thyrotoxicosis, such as toxic nodular goiter, early thyrotoxicosis associated with Hashimoto's thyroiditis or thyrotoxicosis factitia, and toxic adenoma. Some types of hypermetabolic conditions may imitate symptoms of thyrotoxicosis. Examples are a few forms of pheochromocytoma, polycythemia, lymphoma, and leukemias. Pulmonary disease, infection, Parkinsonism, pregnancy, or nephritis may stimulate certain features of pseudothyrotoxicosis.

Though there are various hypotheses about the etiopathogenesis and pathophysiology of GD, the most commonly accepted theory is organ-specific autoimmunity. The treatment of GD is tailor-made to a given patient as there is no single option for cure. The three viable options available for the treatment of GD are antithyroid drugs, ^{131}I radioactive iodine therapy (RAI), and surgical thyroidectomy [1]. The first line of treatment in the majority of cases of GD is aimed at controlling thyrotoxic symptoms for clinical relief and biochemical remission. For this purpose, antithyroid drugs along with beta-blockers and occasionally steroids are started as first-line therapy. There is a difference of opinion as to which of these modalities is best, but institutional guidelines, consensus statements based on geographical parameters, clinician's decision, and patient's choice dictate the treatment algorithm. Antithyroid drugs are widely used for treatment on a long-term basis. About one-third of the patients undergoing long-term antithyroid therapy achieve permanent euthyroidism. Drugs are the preferred initial therapy in children and young adults. Subtotal or Total thyroidectomy is a satisfactory form of therapy if an experienced and/or focused endocrine thyroid surgeon is available. The combined use of antithyroid drugs and iodine makes it possible to prepare patients adequately before surgery with negligible morbidity and mortality. Frequently, surgery is used as a second or third line of treatment when antithyroid drug treatment fails or causes intolerance. Occasionally, surgery is also required for RAI resistant or failed GD [2, 3].

While antithyroid therapy is considered a temporary or symptomatic treatment, RAI and surgery offer permanent or definitive treatment. Currently, most endocrinologists consider RAI the best treatment for adults, and the dosage is calculated based on ^{131}I uptake and gland size. Most patients are cured by one treatment. Hypothyroidism occurs with a constant frequency for many years after therapy, and it is considered an inevitable sequel of ablative therapies.

Thyrotoxicosis in children is best handled initially by antithyroid drug therapy. Surgery may be performed if this therapy does not result in a cure. Treatment with ^{131}I is accepted as an alternative form of treatment by some physicians, especially in children above 15 years of age. Neonatal thyrotoxicosis is a rarity. Antithyroid drugs, propranolol, and iodide may be required for several weeks until maternally-derived antibodies have been metabolized.

The clinician applying any form of the above therapies should take a mature decision and prepare a treatment protocol tailor-made to a given patient based on informed consent, their emotional/ sociopsychological/ financial aspects, and access to the clinician.

Surgical thyroidectomy for GD based on the extent of thyroid tissue removed, includes subtotal, near total and total thyroidectomies. The recent advances in expertise and technology opened up revolutionary options such as sutureless thyroidectomy, robotic thyroidectomy, and endoscopic thyroidectomy. Surgery for GD is challenging due to excess vascularity, risk of thyrotoxic storm and hypocalcemia/ perioperative bleeding risks, and anesthesia related cardiac events. Optimal preoperative preparation and expert surgeon-anesthesiologist combination circumvent these risks in most cases. This chapter specifically emphasizes the indications and role of surgical thyroidectomy for GD. It also includes a detailed discussion on the role, applicability, pros and cons, and various techniques of endoscopic thyroidectomy.

2. Clinical Diagnosis

The diagnosis of Graves' disease can be clinically made in most of the cases based on history, symptoms, and classical signs. In 80-90% of cases, the clinical triad of exophthalmopathic eye signs, goiter, and features of hyperthyroidism (vide infra) forms a pathognomonic diagnostic picture (Figure -1a, 1b). Clinical diagnosis becomes difficult in mild disease; early disease; GD coexisting with other diseases; GD in children, the elderly, and peripartum age groups.

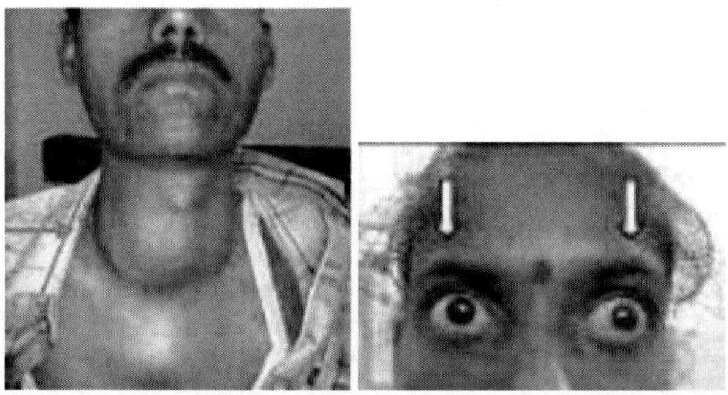

Figure 1. a) Diffuse goiter; b) bilateral exophthalmos.

3. Management of Graves' Disease

Three principal options for the treatment of Graves' disease are blocking of hormone synthesis by antithyroid drugs (ATD), functional destruction of the thyroid by radioiodine (RAI), and partial or total ablation by surgical thyroidectomy. None of these treatments are ideal and universally indicated for all the patients.

At the outset, after diagnosis (clinical and biochemical) of GD, the goals of any treatment are: 1) Prompt control of disease manifestations; 2) Return to and maintenance of euthyroidism; 3) Minimal morbidity and mortality; 4) Reasonable expenses; 5) Long term cure with least chances of recurrence. In the following sections, we discuss them in detail with specific emphasis on the role of surgical thyroidectomy for GD.

3.1. Role of Surgery for Graves' Disease

The technique of general anesthesia, patient position, the surgical technique of open thyroidectomy, general complications, and follow-up management is discussed exhaustively in many textbooks in the literature. Thus, we excluded/ under-addressed the above issues and opted for a non-traditional approach of detailed discussion of the practical issues in surgical management, sharing our experience and recent advances in endoscopic thyroidectomy. To address this intriguing topic, we subdivided it into a few pertinent questions and attempted to answer them in subsequent paragraphs.

1. Indications for surgical thyroidectomy
2. Preoperative preparation
3. Recommended Surgical extent
4. Types and techniques of surgery
5. Details of surgical management
6. Advantages of surgery
7. Disadvantages/ complications of surgery
8. Influence of surgery on Graves' Ophthalmopathy.

3.1.1. Indications for Surgical Thyroidectomy

The definitive treatment in the form of surgical thyroidectomy is indicated for GD in the following circumstances:

1. Coincident malignant nodules
2. Associated Ophthalmopathy
3. Large volume thyroid gland
4. Presence of compressive symptoms
5. Substernal thyroid extension
6. Contraindications for the use of Radio-iodine, e.g., pregnancy, children
7. Intolerance to anti-thyroid drugs
8. Presence of a dominant nodule
9. Recurrence after RAI therapy
10. Marine Lenhart Syndrome
11. Very High TSAb (Thyroid Stimulating antibody)
12. Chronic smoking
13. Patient preference

The surgical indications can be further refined into absolute and relative indications:

The absolute indications for surgical thyroidectomy are:

1. Graves' disease with documented suspicious or malignant nodules (~20% of thyroid nodules in Graves' disease are thyroid cancers)
2. Pregnant patients:
   - Not readily controlled by anti-thyroid drugs
   - Serious allergic reactions to drugs
3. Patients intolerant or unresponsive to anti-thyroid drugs
4. Local compressive symptoms: Pain or dysphagia

The relative indications for surgical thyroidectomy are:

1. Patients with poor compliance to drugs; there are higher chances of hypothyroidism after RAI ablation than surgical ablation
2. Desirous of rapid control of symptoms (RAI has a 6 week to 6 month latency period)
3. Patients with severe manifestations of Graves' Ophthalmopathy
4. Large volume goiters and relatively low RAI uptake
5. Psychologically or mentally incompetent patients
6. Those who are unable to maintain long term follow up.

3.1.2. Preoperative Preparation for Surgery

It is vital and desirable to attain preoperative euthyroidism to avoid intra or post-operative thyroid storm and facilitate safe surgery. Apart from general surgical preparation and ensuring anesthetic fitness, the following steps are used to achieve this objective

1. Combination of Thionamides + Iodine with or without beta blockers
2. Most commonly, a titration method is used
3. It is desirable to render the patient both clinically and chemically euthyroid
4. Propranolol to control clinical features of hyperthyroidism, which is continued postoperatively and tapered over 7-10 days. In diabetic and asthmatic patients, cardioselective beta blockers are used.

5. Some centers use the Block and Treat regimen, wherein a titrated combination of thionamides and levothyroxine is used. But, it has only a limited role in regular practice.
6. Some centers use iodine in the form of Lugol's Iodine (LI) or saturated solution of potassium iodide (SSKI). But iodine has varying effects depending on its length of administration. It Inhibits the release of T4 & T3 from the thyroid: in its early administration. The onset of action occurs within 24 hours with maximum effect after 2 weeks of use, but its benefit is temporary. Large doses or prolonged usage were found to worsen hyperthyroidism. Thus, LI with a dose of 5-10 drops thrice a day or SSKI of 1 drop thrice a day is given for two weeks prior to surgery along with thionamides with or without propranolol. It was found that the thyroid gland becomes less vascular and firmer and thus rendering surgery less complicated. But this benefit is only theoretical in most of the cases.
7. Lithium carbonate is used in ATD non-responders and refractory cases.

3.1.3. Extent of Surgery

The usually performed surgeries for GD can be classified as Subtotal thyroidectomy (STT); Near total thyroidectomy (NTT); Dunhill's procedure (total lobectomy + contralateral partial lobectomy); and Total thyroidectomy (TT).

Near total thyroidectomy and total thyroidectomy are technically different, but both are similar in terms of outcome. Though the theoretical and published experience suggests lower morbidity due to hypocalcemia or recurrent laryngeal nerve palsy in NTT compared to TT. Dunhill's procedure is not performed universally but is mentioned here for academic purposes. The two most common procedures performed and the see-saw battle of choices is between STT versus TT. There is no consensus on the definition of STT as the remnant of the thyroid gland left over after the procedure is not objectively measurable. There are various definitions based on estimated weight, volume, vascularity, the safety of parathyroid glands, and recurrent laryngeal nerves. The acceptable yet empirical definition of STT is the minimal part of the entire thyroid gland left over as remnants in both trachea-esophageal grooves, ensuring the safety of parathyroid glands and recurrent laryngeal nerves and also remnant adequate enough to maintain euthyroidism. In both these procedures, the risk of long-term hypothyroidism is an issue. While in TT, it is an inevitable and predictable sequel, in STT, it is unpredictable and long-term morbidity as up to 70% of patients undergoing STT end up with hypothyroidism. In one of the large studies reported by Sugino et al., (3), thyroid function was assessed up to three years after STT on 1897 patients. The rate of euthyroidism decreased by 40%, and the rate of hypothyroidism increased by 52% by the third postoperative year. Thus, the risk of hypothyroidism is inversely proportional to the remnant size and the longer follow-up duration.

At the other end of the spectrum, the risk of recurrent hyperthyroidism is also higher in STT than TT. It is obvious that the chances of recurrence after TT is negligible as we are removing all macroscopic thyroid tissue leading to its total ablation. Rarely, any inadvertently left surgical remnants or embryologically segregated ectopic thyroid foci may lead to recurrent hyperthyroidism as the underlying etiopathology is active. But, the chances of this depend on surgeon's expertise and experience. Various studies showed that chances of recurrent hyperthyroidism are another unpredictable morbidity of STT with as much as 16% after 30 years of follow-up. The risk of recurrence is directly proportional to remnant size. It is estimated that a remnant size of more than 10 grams significantly increases the risk of recurrences and each 1 gram increase in remnant size decreases the rate of hypothyroidism by 10%.

3.1.4. Types and Techniques Of Surgery

The recent advances and accumulated experience over decades have opened up several options and surgical techniques. Based on the access route, thyroidectomy can be classified as follows:

1. Open Conventional thyroidectomy
    - Cervical
    - Thoracic (for associated large intrathoracic/ retrosternal extensions)
        - Sternotomy
        - Thoracotomy
            - Anterior
            - Anterolateral
            - Posterolateral
2. Suture less thyroidectomy

3. Endoscopic thyroidectomy
   - MIVAT (minimal invasive video assisted thyroidectomy)
   - With Gas insufflation
   - Gasless technique
   - Axillary, chest wall routes
   - Thoracoscopic
   - Novel routes – Trans-oral, retroauricular.

3.2. Details of Surgical Management

3.2.1. Open Thyroidectomy

Thyroid surgery has been performed since ancient times and has followed many steps of evolution to reach the present times of endoscopic surgery. Conventional open thyroidectomies are effective, safe, well-tolerated, and time tested but leave an evident scar in the exposed part of the body, which can occasionally be cosmetically unacceptable in some cases. Subtotal thyroidectomy (STT) is a well established and optimal form of ablative therapy for Graves' disease, provided the patient has been suitably prepared for surgery. STT is widely practiced by surgeons around the globe, especially by general and otolaryngology surgeons. In competent hands, the risk of hypoparathyroidism or recurrent nerve damage is under 1%, and the discomfort and transient disability attendant upon surgery may be an acceptable price to pay for the rapid relief from this disease. In some clinics, it is the therapy of choice for most young male adults, especially if a trial of antithyroid drugs has failed. Total thyroidectomy may be preferred in patients with serious eye disease or high TRAb levels, in order to help the eye disease and to keep down the incidence of recurrence [4–8].

As with other effective methods available, it is necessary for the physician and the patient to decide on the form of therapy most suitable for the case at hand. Because of the potential but unproved risks of 131-I therapy, it is not always possible to make an entirely rational choice; the physician's and patient's fears and prejudices will often enter into the decision. Surgery is clearly indicated in certain patients. Among these are (1) patients who have not responded to prolonged antithyroid drug therapy or who develop toxic reactions to the drug and, for whatever reason, are unsuitable for 131-I therapy; (2) patients with large volume goiter, which frequently do not regress adequately after 131-I therapy; and (3) patients with thyroid nodules that raise suspicion of carcinoma. Stocker et al., have reviewed the problem of nodules in Graves' glands [9]. They found that 12% of Graves' patients had cold defects on the scan, and half of these were referred for surgery. Six of 22, representing 2% of all Graves' patients, 15% of patients with cold nodules, 25% of patients with palpable nodules, and 27% of those going to surgery, had papillary cancer in the location corresponding to the cold defect. Of these patients, one had metastasis to bone, and two required multiple treatments with radioiodine. These authors argue for evaluating patients with a thyroid scintigram and further diagnostic evaluation of cold defects. Subtotal or near total thyroidectomy is often the treatment of choice for patients with amiodarone induced thyrotoxicosis since the response to ATDs is typically poor, and RAIU cannot be given [10]. Surgery may also have a place in the therapy of older patients with thyroid storm and/or cardio-respiratory failure, who do not respond rapidly to intensive medical therapy [11].

3.2.2. Endoscopic Thyroidectomy (ET) or Minimal Access Thyroidectomy (MAT)

A glance at the history of thyroidectomy reveals how it was developed by pioneer endocrine and thyroid surgeons through various stages till the present era of minimal access surgery [12]. Endoscopic thyroidectomy (ET) has rapidly transformed from a fantasy into reality. Ever since the onset of the laparoscopic era in the early 1980s, minimal access surgery occupies the major share of operation theater lists in most surgical disciplines. Increasing confidence and experience in laparoscopic surgical skills have permeated into endocrine surgery after the demonstration of endoscopic subtotal parathyroidectomy and thyroidectomy in 1996 by Gagner [13]. This was extended to thyroid nodules in 1997 by Huscher et al., who employed a skin incision at the anterior border of sternocleidomastoid [14]. In the recent past, more centers are performing ET in increasing numbers, mostly in Western and affluent Asian countries. Minimally access surgery of the neck was first developed for the management of thyroid and parathyroid disorders. ET is in the phase of evolution. Though open conventional thyroidectomy is still the favored approach worldwide, a plethora of Endoscopic Thyroidectomy (ET) techniques ranging from totally endoscopic, video-assisted, trans-axillary, and chest-wall procedures have been already employed [12, 15–18]. Even novel approaches such as thoracoscopic, robotic, trans-oral, and post-auricular routes have been explored [19–23]. Figures 3 to 10 illustrate few of these approaches. Though none of them are validated universally, the majority favors chest-wall and trans-axillary approaches.

The objectives of any ET technique are better cosmesis, lesser pain, lower morbidity, and feasibility in patients with co-morbidities. Most of the available ET techniques fulfill cosmetic and pain aspects but fail to address the latter two factors. Based on the use of carbon dioxide gas insufflation (CO_2), ET may be broadly divided into gas dependent and gasless techniques. In an effort to lessen the adverse aesthetic effects of conventional open surgical techniques and gas-dependent ET techniques, gasless ET techniques have evolved.

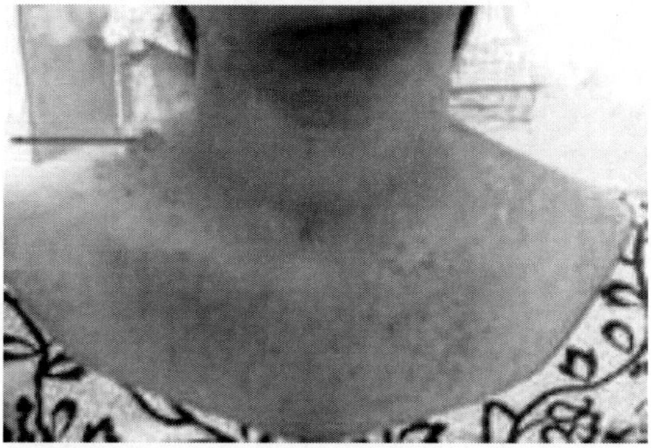

Figure 2. Skin rashes with ATD.

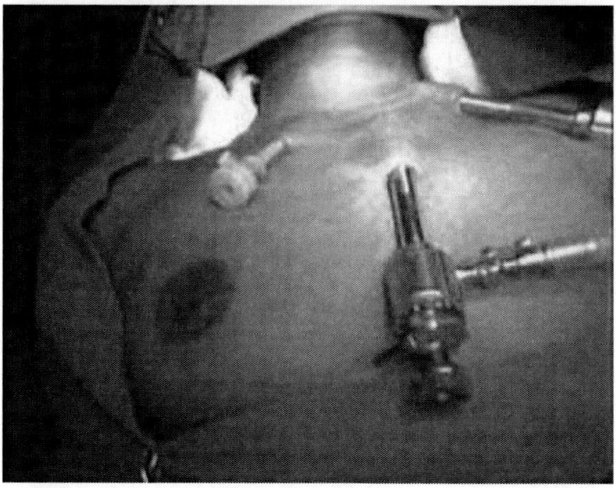

Figure 3. Trans chest wall endoscopic thyroidectomy – port placements.

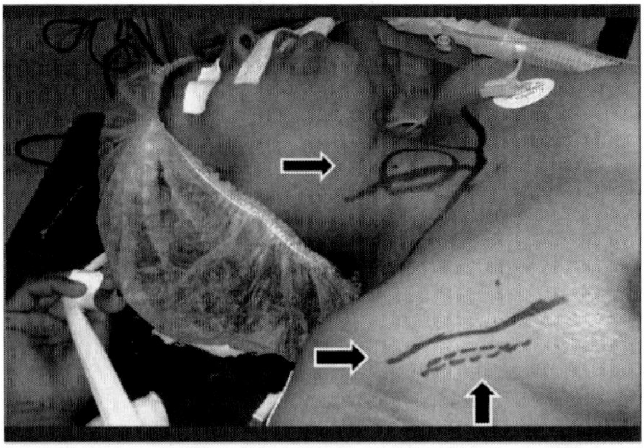

Figure 4. Endoscopic transaxillary thyroidectomy – preoperative surgical markings.

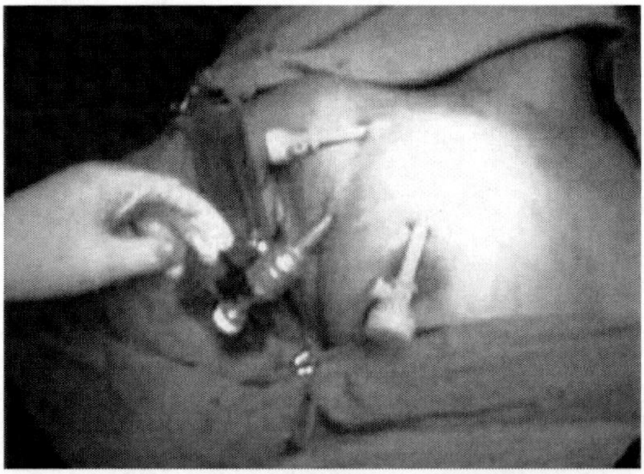

Figure 5. Trans axillary (gas based) endoscopic thyroidectomy.

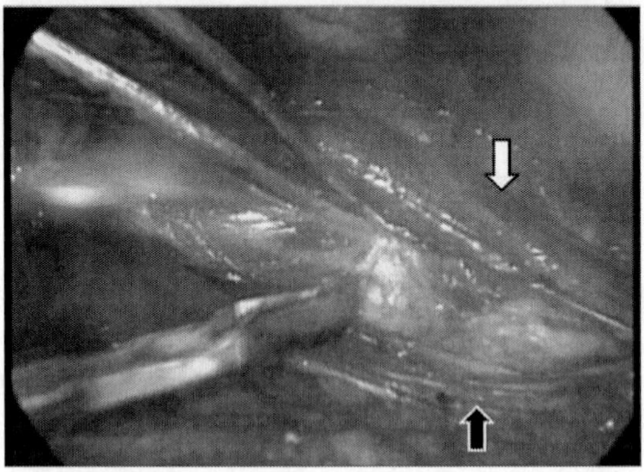

Figure 6. Intraoperative view of transaxillary endoscopic thyroidectomy.

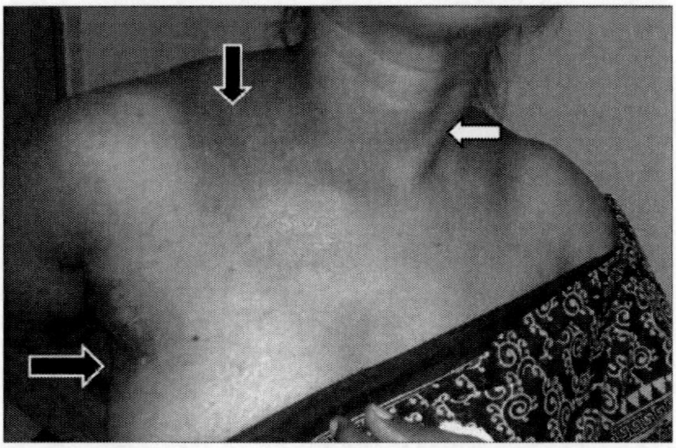

Figure 7. post operative scarless neck and good cosmesis after transaxillary thyroidectomy.

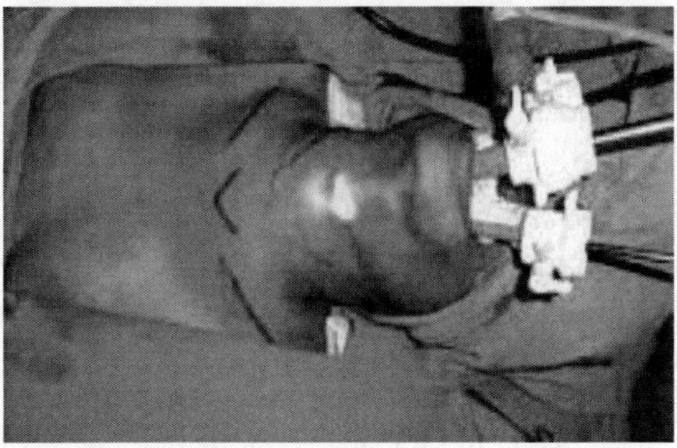

Figure 8. Transoral thyroidectomy – port placement through lower gingival sulcus.

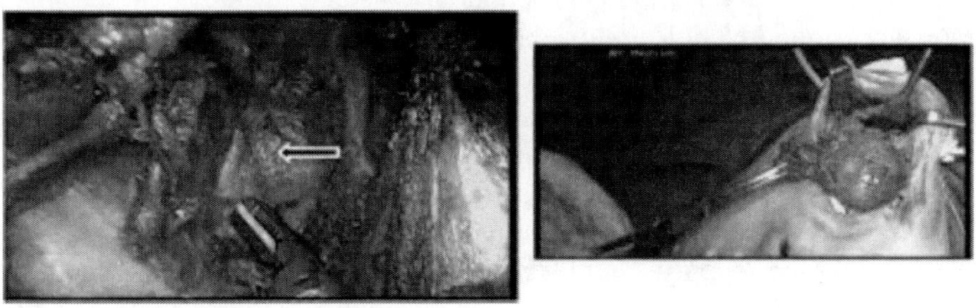

Figure 9. Transoral thyroidectomy; Intraoperative view, Specimen extraction.

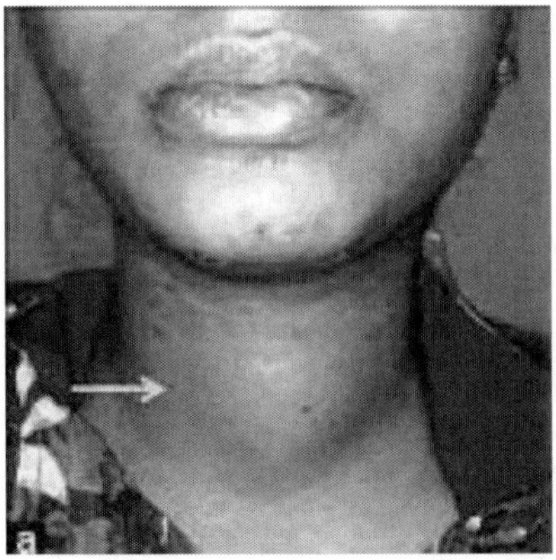

Figure 10. Postoperative excellent cosmesis after transoral thyroidectomy.

All the ET techniques necessitate the creation of a subcutaneous working space by using external or internal maneuvers. The commonest internal manoeuver is gas insufflation at a predetermined pressure. Various gases tried in both animal, and human subjects are carbon dioxide, nitrogen, nitrous oxide, helium, air, krypton, and argon. The CO2 insufflation proved to be the best option due to its high solubility, low cost, and non-combustibility [24]. Due to the lack of pre-existing anatomical cavity in the region, the creation of a new space requires the use of gas insufflation pressure as high as 20 mm Hg or prolonged low pressure insufflation. Various animal studies have been performed to study the hemodynamic and metabolic changes at different pressures of CO2 insufflation in endoscopic neck surgery. CO2 insufflation pressure of < 8 mm Hg is found safe in many studies [25–27]. When higher pressure is required, a level lower than 15 mm Hg is recommended, and the insufflation duration should be reduced to limit the complications [28, 29]. Ryoichi et al., used a long subcutaneous dissector to create a subcutaneous space. After dissection, an insufflation pressure of 6 mm Hg was high enough to maintain the surgical space and also low enough to avoid significant CO2 absorption through the subcutaneous tissue [30]. An anterior cervical approach using carbondioxide insufflation pressure (CIP) of 10 mm Hg was described by Gagner et al., [13] A breast approach for ET with a low CIP of 4 to 6 mm of Hg was reported by Park et al., [25]. We used carbon dioxide insufflation pressure (CIP) of 12 to 14 mm Hg till the creation of working space and CIP of 8 to 10 mm Hg for maintenance of the created working space. Complications unique to endoscopic neck surgery are mostly related to insufflation of CO2 gas and CO2 diffusion into the body tissues and spaces, which can lead to devastating consequences. Complications due to CO2 may range from severe hypercarbia, subcutaneous emphysema, tension pneumothorax, pneumomediastinum, CO2 embolism to cardiac arrhythmias and myocardial suppression. Excessive exposure to CO2 can lead to diffusion and absorption of gas through available tissue planes to cause severe hypercarbia and other complications. Moreover, massive subcutaneous emphysema may act as a reservoir for continuous CO2 absorption leading to pneumomediastinum and pneumothorax [31]. Murdock et al., showed an operative time of > 200 minutes and ETCO2 of >50 mm Hg as independent risk factors for hypercarbia, subcutaneous emphysema, pneumothorax, and pneumomediastinum [26]. Glottlieb et al., reported massive subcutaneous emphysema with severe hypercarbia and refractory supraventricular tachycardia in the case of endoscopic parathyroidectomy [32]. Improved anesthetic and perioperative management were proposed to reduce gas related complications [31]. CO2 absorption can be estimated with reasonable accuracy using indirect calorimetry during surgery. Continuous ETCO2 monitoring with appropriate ventilatory adjustments ensures safe surgery, though ET is not recommended as a routine procedure [33]. Hypercarbia and acidosis can be controlled by enhancing the ventilation rate and minute ventilation. Some investigators suggested routine use of arterial blood gas (ABG) analysis for better monitoring of CO2 levels [34]. Thus, in any gas dependent ET technique, a CO2 insufflation pressure (CIP) of 10 to 12 mm Hg for creating working space and 6 to 8 mm Hg for maintaining space during endoscopic thyroidectomy appears to be optimal. A protocol based on proper patient selection, intraoperative monitoring, and intermittent CO2 desufflation is desirable to ensure safe surgery with minimal gas-related complications.

In the gasless technique through the transaxillary route, the incision taken in the axilla remains hidden beneath the clothes. Due to a natural plane, the creation of the subpectoral space and its continuation in the subplatysmal plane in the neck is easy. The thyroid bed is reached through two heads of the sternocleidomastoid muscle (SCM) without the need to divide or split the strap muscles. Throughout the procedure, an assistant retracts the sternal head of SCM along with strap muscles anteromedially. As the space is created after dissection, it does not require carbon dioxide gas (CO_2), thus preventing gas-related morbidity. Synergistic use of the naked eye and magnified monitor vision ensures accurate identification and preservation of vital structures like RLN and PTG. In this technique, the apparent disadvantage is increased area of dissection in the infraclavicular region. As the OS visualizes the operative field horizontally through the axillary incision, it becomes challenging to reach the opposite thyroid lobe. Thus, the excision of the opposite lobe needs another incision in the contralateral axilla. To hold the telescope without a fulcrum is another task for CA. Despite these shortcomings, the end result is gratifying for the patient and surgeon with a virtually scarless thyroidectomy.

The gas dependent techniques can cause serious hypercarbia associated complications such as subcutaneous emphysema, mediastinal emphysema, cardiac arrhythmias and even death in a few cases. Especially, patients with comorbid conditions such as hypertension, diabetes, and chronic obstructive airway disease are susceptible to complications. These complications are related to CO_2 insufflation pressures, length of surgery, susceptibility and comorbid conditions of the patient. Lower CO_2 insufflation pressures, intensive end tidal CO_2 monitoring ($EtCO_2$), intra-operative arterial blood gas analysis (ABG), intermittent desufflation, shorter operative times, proper patient selection have been recommended to counter these gas-related complications. On the contrary, gasless techniques are very safe as it nullifies the whole gamut of gas-related morbidity. Thus, even patients with well to moderately controlled comorbidities can be taken up for surgery which allows longer operative times with extra safety. It also reduces the cost of intensive $EtCO_2$ and ABG monitoring used for gas dependent techniques. The only practical disadvantage of gasless over gas dependent technique is inadequate operative space, which can be compensated by proper retraction by AS and synergistic naked eye and camera vision of thyroid area.

3.2.2.1. Operative Principles of ET

We attempted to describe the basic surgical principles of any ET technique in ten steps in chronological order in the following sections.

- *Access, ports, and operative space creation*: Surgical access can be broadly classified as cervical and extracervical routes. Within extracervical routes, TA, CW, and AB approaches are more frequently practiced. It is still early to comment on the superiority of one technique over the other. Usually, a 10 mm camera port and two 5 mm working ports are used with an additional port optionally.
- Irrespective of the access route, operative space (OS) has to be created in contrast to the natural OS in abdomen or pleural cavity. We create OS through a combination of blunt and sharp subcutaneous or subpectoral fascial dissection with long hemostats, balloon inflation, and diathermy dissection under vision. This dissection is continued in

subplatysmal plane of the neck beyond the clavicle. This latter dissection is done up to the level of thyroid cartilage and over the ipsilateral thyroid lobe.

- *Reaching thyroid gland in visceral space of neck*: In ET, similar to open thyroidectomy, the thyroid goiter (TG) can be approached through midline between strap muscles or lateral approach between strap muscle and sternocleidomastoid (SCM) muscle. This lateral approach is especially useful in ET as it is an avascular plane, avoids anterior jugular veins, and aids in direct control of the middle thyroid vein. With diathermy, the deep fascia over this plane is incised and SCM is retracted. Lateral one-third of strap muscles can be cut for extra space. The middle thyroid vein is controlled with clips.
- *Mobilization of the thyroid gland*: Deep-to-deep cervical fascia, the avascular plane between thyroid lobe and carotid sheath, is further opened up till prevertebral fascia. Pretracheal fascia over the thyroid lobe is teased close to TG and it is rotated medially. This dissection continues till the lateral part of the superior thyroid pedicle is visualized.
- *Control of superior thyroid pedicle*: Strap muscle overlying the TG is retracted and if needed its lateral one-third is cut. Once superior pedicle blood vessels are visualized, they must be skeletonized, teasing away the pretracheal fascia and strap muscle fibers with bipolar diathermy. The skeletonized pedicle blood vessels are individually double clipped on the proximal side and single clipped toward TG. They are divided to devascularize TG superiorly.
- *Control of inferior thyroid pedicle*: With the combination of blunt and sharp dissection assisted by diathermy, the trachea below the ipsilateral isthmolobar junction is visualized. The multiple inferior thyroid veins (ITVs) should be skeletonized from the medial to the lateral side. ITVs are individually clipped and divided. Before dividing lateral most ITV, it is mandatory to differentiate it from recurrent laryngeal nerve (RLN) as it courses parallel to them. If in doubt, lateral ITV should be divided after the demonstration of RLN only. However, with endoscopic magnification, it is not as difficult to differentiate ITV from RLN as in open surgery.
- *Identification of recurrent laryngeal nerve (RLN)*: As ET is usually performed for smaller goiters, RLN lies in the normal location in the majority of cases. It courses in trachea-esophageal groove between

the branches of ITA. With endoscopic magnification, RLN is seen very clearly seen as a white string-like structure with a vasa nervosum accompanying it, posterior to TG. Low-amperage diathermy current is employed at least 2 mm away from RLN to divide vascular structures. RLN is followed up, until its entry at the lower border of inferior pharyngeal constrictor.

- *Parathyroid glands (PTGs)*: Thorough anatomical and embryological knowledge along with adequate experience in thyroid surgery is mandatory to identify PTG. They should be looked for in usual anatomical locations. Superior PTG, which is the most constant, is located posterosuperior to RLN in more than 80% of individuals. Capsular dissection close to the capsule of TG with meticulous hemostasis using bipolar diathermy is done to preserve PTG. Inferior PTG is located antero-inferior to RLN over the inferior pole of thyroid, which is dissected and preserved similar to superior PTG.
- *Ligament of Berry*: Division of the posterior suspensory ligament of the thyroid also known as the ligament of Berry is the penultimate step of ET. After identification of RLN over its entire course, the ligament of Berry is divided close to TG and away from RLN using bipolar diathermy, as it is a vascular structure.
- *Separation of TG from thyroid bed*: The only attachment of TG in neck after prior steps is flimsy, hypovascular areolar tissue between TG and tracheal perichondrium. It is dissected with sharp dissection using scissors after elevation of TG off the trachea.
- *Specimen extraction*: Similar procedural steps are repeated on the contralateral side for total thyroidectomy. The thyroidectomy specimen is retrieved from the camera port under vision, after enlarging the incision by 1–2 cm. Placement of drain is optional after checking the thyroid bed for hemostasis.

3.3. Advantages of Surgical Management

1. Rapid euthyroidism with immediate cure of disease (in RAI, euthyroidism is achieved with a delay of 4-6 months)
2. Avoids long-term risks of RAI
3. Provides tissue for histologic examination
4. Apparently easier titration of Thyroid hormone replacement

5. Avoids the use of steroids for associated TAO (Thyroid associated Ophthalmopathy)
6. Complication rates are low in High Volume centers with experienced endocrine surgeons
7. Safe in pregnancy and lactation
8. Avoids RAI induced Hyperparathyroidism (a rare event).

3.4. Disadvantages/Complications of Total Thyroidectomy

A well indicated, well planned, and well executed total thyroidectomy by an experienced surgical-anesthetic team has negligible (less than 1% of complications) and near zero mortality risk. For academic purposes and as ideal management is not always possible, the list of disadvantages (both technical and non-technical) is mentioned below:

1. One-time surgical management is more expensive than RAI or ATD
2. Wound complications such as infections, seroma, cervical hematoma
3. Damage to external branch of superior laryngeal nerve (EBSLN): about 1% chances (voice fatigue and loss of high pitch quality)
4. Damage to the recurrent laryngeal nerve (RLN): hoarseness of voice, anesthesia of supralaryngeal mucosa
5. Risk of permanent Vocal cord paralysis: 0-2%
6. Risk of Temporary vocal cord palsy (10-50%)
7. Risk of Permanent Hypoparathyroidism (less than 2%)

The three main complications of thyroidectomy are hemorrhage, hypocalcemia and voice change.

3.4.1. Hemorrhage

Hemorrhage: Bleeding in the neck after thyroid surgery can lead to compromise of the airway and it is therefore a potentially very serious complication. The overall incidence of bleeding in the neck reported in the literature is around 1.2% of cases and although thyroid surgeons would probably feel that patients with thyrotoxicosis and large multinodular goiters are more likely to bleed postoperatively than those with thyroid carcinoma, this is not borne out in the literature. Meticulous attention to detail at the operation with careful identification and control of the main vessels supplying and draining the thyroid will minimize the risk of bleeding. The main sources of bleeding are strap muscles, anterior jugular veins, vascular pedicles and rarely secondary hemorrhage.

3.4.2. Post Thyroidectomy Hypocalcemia

Malfunction of the parathyroid glands following thyroid surgery is explained on the basis of their anatomical and vascular relationship with the thyroid gland. The parathyroid glands are most commonly close to the posterior and lateral aspect of the thyroid gland and share their blood supply with the thyroid. It is therefore incumbent upon the thyroid surgeon to accurately identify the parathyroid glands at the time of the operation and to preserve and protect them when possible. The technique of capsular dissection of the thyroid, whereby the blood supply to the thyroid gland is secured very close to the edge of the gland, as opposed to the main trunk of the superior or inferior thyroid arteries, should minimize devascularization of the parathyroid glands.

3.4.3. Voice Change

Voice change and dysphagia can occur after surgery to the thyroid gland. Dysphagia is reported in up to 1.4% of patients and should be mentioned in the preoperative discussions [2]. Voice change is reported in the literature as being permanent in about 1% of the patients due to recurrent laryngeal nerve damage on one side and in approximately 3.7% due to damage to the superior laryngeal nerve. Damage from nerve injuries can be reduced to a minimum if the nerves are routinely located during the operation and traced to the inlet of the lower pharyngeal constrictor muscle. Unipolar diathermy should be avoided in close proximity to the nerve and care should be taken to look for evidence of a non-recurrent laryngeal nerve.

3.5. Role of Surgical Thyroidectomy in Graves' Associated Ophthalmopathy (GAO)

Graves' disease (GD) is an organ-specific autoimmune thyroid disease caused primarily by a thyroid-stimulating autoantibody (TSAb) acting on the TSH receptor of the thyrocyte membrane [35, 36]. The natural history of ophthalmopathic exophthalmos is divided into progressive, plateau and resolution phases. Occasionally, GAO can undergo gradual spontaneous resolution. These phases have variable duration and alter with thyroid functional status. GAE is an objectively and reproducibly measurable component of GAO with exophthalmometry. The most common method of its accurate measurement is by Hertel's exophthalmometry [37]. The upper limits of exophthalmos vary between different ethnic groups with 18 mm for Asians, 20 mm for Caucasians and 22 mm for Africans [38]. Vasanth kumar et al., reported that the ethnic race of South Indians had a maximum PFH compared to Caucasians and Mongolians [39]. In one of our previously published study, we showed that a mean palpabrel fissure height (PFH) of 10.37 mm, after regression of GAE (from 12.67 mm) (Figure 11). The improvement was statistically significant on *t* test at 0.04. GAE regresses in 73% of cases at 1 year with significant symptomatic relief, after thyroidectomy [40]. Abrupt alteration in thyroid functional status can be complicated with exacerbation of GAO, often with loss of sight in severe cases [41]. In two of our cases, GAO had self-limiting mild exacerbation at 4 and 6 weeks respectively, in spite of maintaining postoperative euthyroidism. With available evidence from published literature, Total thyroidectomy appears to be ideal management for GAO with a better prognostic impact than RAI [42].

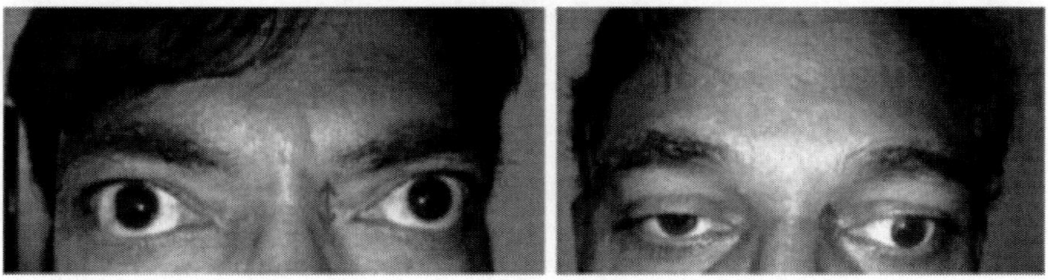

Figure 11. Bilateral regression of GAE at last follow-up of 30 months. [Markers placed for PFH comparison before (*left*) and after (*right*) surgery].

References

[1] Törring O, Tallstedt L, Wallin G, Lundell G, Ljunggren JG, Taube A, Sääf M, Hamberger B. Graves' hyperthyroidism: treatment with antithyroid drugs, surgery, or radioiodine--a prospective, randomized study. Thyroid Study Group. *J Clin Endocrinol Metab*. 1996 Aug;81(8):2986–93.

[2] Bhargav PRK, Amar V, Uday SK. Recurrent Graves' disease after successful radioiodine therapy induced hypothyroidism: A rare occurrence. *World Journal of Endocrine Surgery*. 2011;3(3):134–6.

[3] Sugino K, Ito K, Nagahama M, Kitagawa W, Shibuya H, Ito K. Surgical management of Graves' disease - 10-Year prospective trial at a single institution. *Endocr J*. 2008;55(1):161–7.

[4] Klementschitsch P, Shen K liang, Kaplan EL. Reemergence of Thyroidectomy as Treatment for Graves' Disease. *Surgical Clinics of North America*. 1979 Feb;59(1):35–44.
[5] Palit TK, Miller CC, Miltenburg DM. The efficacy of thyroidectomy for Graves' disease: A meta-analysis. *Journal of Surgical Research*. 2000;90(2):161–5.
[6] Winsa B, Rastad J, Akerstrom G, Johansson H, Westermark K, Karlsson FA. Retrospective evaluation of subtotal and total thyroidectomy in Graves' disease with and without endocrine ophthalmopathy. *Eur J Endocrinol*. 1995;132(4):406–12.
[7] Sundaresh V, Brito JP, Wang Z, Prokop LJ, Stan MN, Murad MH, Bahn RS. Comparative Effectiveness of Therapies for Graves' Hyperthyroidism: A Systematic Review and Network Meta-Analysis. *J Clin Endocrinol Metab*. 2013 Sep;98(9):3671–7.
[8] Hamilton RD, Mayberry WE, McConahey WM, Hanson KC. Ophthalmopathy of Graves' disease: a comparison between patients treated surgically and patients treated with radioiodide. *Mayo Clin Proc*. 1967;42(12):812–8.
[9] Stocker DJ, Foster SS, Solomon BL, Shriver CD, Burch HB. Thyroid cancer yield in patients with Graves' disease selected for surgery on the basis of cold scintiscan defects. *Thyroid*. 2002;12(4).
[10] Bogazzi F, Miccoli P, Berti P, Cosci C, Brogioni S, Aghini-Lombardi F, Materazzi G, Bartalena L, Pinchera A, Braverman LE, Martino E. Preparation with iopanoic acid rapidly controls thyrotoxicosis in patients with amiodarone-induced thyrotoxicosis before thyroidectomy. *Surgery*. 2002 Dec;132(6):1114–8.
[11] Scholz GH, Hagemann E, Arkenau C, Engelmann L, Lamesch P, Schreiter D, Schoenfelder M, Olthoff D, Paschke R. Is There a Place for Thyroidectomy in Older Patients with Thyrotoxic Storm and Cardiorespiratory Failure? *Thyroid*. 2003 Oct;13(10):933–40.
[12] Rogers-Stevane J, Kauffman GL. A Historical Perspective on Surgery of the Thyroid and Parathyroid Glands. *Otolaryngol Clin North Am*. 2008 Dec;41(6):1059–67.
[13] Gagner M, Inabnet WB. Endoscopic Thyroidectomy for Solitary Thyroid Nodules. *Thyroid*. 2001 Feb;11(2):161–3.
[14] Lirici MM, Hüscher CSG, Chiodini S, Napolitano C, Recher A. Endoscopic right thyroid lobectomy. *Surg Endosc*. 1997 Aug 15;11(8):877–877.
[15] Inabnet III WB, Jacob BP, Gagner M. Minimally invasive endoscopic thyroidectomy by a cervical approach. *Surg Endosc*. 2003 Nov 1;17(11):1808–11.
[16] Ikeda Y, Takami H, Sasaki Y, Takayama J, Niimi M, Kan S. Clinical Benefits in Endoscopic Thyroidectomy by the Axillary Approach. *J Am Coll Surg*. 2003 Feb;196(2):189–95.
[17] Miccoli P, Bellantone R, Mourad M, Walz M, Raffaelli M, Berti P. Minimally Invasive Video-assisted Thyroidectomy: Multiinstitutional Experience. *World J Surg*. 2002 Aug 1;26(8):972–5.
[18] Yeung GHC. Endoscopic Thyroid Surgery Today: A Diversity of Surgical Strategies. *Thyroid*. 2002 Aug;12(8):703–6.

[19] Shimazu K, Shiba E, Tamaki Y, Takiguchi S, Taniguchi E, Ohashi S, Noguchi S. Endoscopic Thyroid Surgery Through the Axillo-Bilateral-Breast Approach. *Surg Laparosc Endosc Percutan Tech*. 2003 Jun;13(3):196–201.

[20] Witzel K, von Rahden BHA, Kaminski C, Stein HJ. Transoral access for endoscopic thyroid resection. *Surg Endosc.* 2008 Aug 28;22(8):1871–5.

[21] Bhargav PRK, Bhagat SD, Kishan Rao B, Murthy SGK, Amar V. Combined Cervical and Video-assisted Thoracoscopic Thyroidectomy (CAVATT): A Simplified and Innovative Approach for Goiter with Posterior Mediastinal Extension. *Indian Journal of Surgery*. 2010 Aug 16;72(4):336–8.

[22] Kang SW, Park JH, Jeong JS, Lee CR, Park S, Lee SH, Jeong JJ, Nam KH, Chung WY, Park CS. Prospects of Robotic Thyroidectomy Using a Gasless, Transaxillary Approach for the Management of Thyroid Carcinoma. *Surg Laparosc Endosc Percutan Tech*. 2011 Aug;21(4):223–9.

[23] Lee KE, Kim HY, Park WS, Choe JH, Kwon MR, Oh SK, Youn YK. Postauricular and Axillary Approach Endoscopic Neck Surgery: A New Technique. *World J Surg*. 2009 Apr 7;33(4):767–72.

[24] Menes T, Spivak H. Laparoscopy Searching for the proper insufflation gas. *Surg Endosc*. 2000 Nov 1;14(11):1050–6.

[25] Park YL, Han WK, Bae WG. 100 Cases of Endoscopic Thyroidectomy. *Surg Laparosc Endosc Percutan Tech*. 2003 Feb;13(1):20–5.

[26] Murdock C. Risk factors for hypercarbia, subcutaneous emphysema, pneumothorax, and pneumomediastinum during laparoscopy. *Obstetrics & Gynecology.* 2000 May;95(5):704–9.

[27] Duncan TD, Rashid Q, Speights F, Ejeh I. Endoscopic transaxillary approach to the thyroid gland: our early experience. *Surg Endosc*. 2007 Dec 4;21(12):2166–71.

[28] Chantawibul S, Lokechareonlarp S, Pokawatana C. Total Video Endoscopic Thyroidectomy by an Axillary Approach. *Journal of Laparoendoscopic & Advanced Surgical Techniques*. 2003 Oct;13(5):295–9.

[29] Rubino F, Pamoukian VN, Zhu JF, Deutsch H, Inabnet WB, Gagner M. Endoscopic endocrine neck surgery with carbon dioxide insufflation: The effect on intracranial pressure in a large animal model. *Surgery*. 2000 Dec;128(6):1035–42.

[30] Ochiai R, Takeda J, Noguchi J, Ohgami M, Ishii S. Subcutaneous Carbon Dioxide Insufflation Does Not Cause Hypercarbia During Endoscopic Thyroidectomy. *Anesth Analg*. 2000 Mar;90(3):760.

[31] Doctor NH, Hussain Z. Bilateral pneumothorax associated with laparoscopy. *Anaesthesia*. 1973 Jan;28(1):75–81.

[32] Gottlieb A, Sprung J, Zheng XM, Gagner M. Massive Subcutaneous Emphysema and Severe Hypercarbia in a Patient During Endoscopic Transcervical Parathyroidectomy Using Carbon Dioxide Insufflation. *Anesth Analg*. 1997 May;84(5):1154–6.

[33] Wahba RWM, Mamazza J. Ventilatory requirements during laparoscopic cholecystectomy. *Canadian Journal of Anaesthesia*. 1993 Mar;40(3):206–10.

[34] Bellantone R. Arterial PCO2 and Cardiovascular Function During Endoscopic Neck Surgery With Carbon Dioxide Insufflation. *Archives of Surgery*. 2001 Jul 1;136(7):822.

[35] Smith BR, McLachlan SM, Furmaniak J. Autoantibodies to the Thyrotropin Receptor. *Endocr Rev*. 1988 Feb;9(1):106–21.

[36] Amino N, Yuasa T, Yabu Y, Miyai K, Kumahara Y. Exophthalmos in Autoimmune Thyroid Disease*. *J Clin Endocrinol Metab*. 1980 Dec;51(6):1232–4.

[37] Mourits MP, Lombardo SHC, Sluijs FA van der, Fenton S. Reliability of exophthalmos measurement and the exophthalmometry value distribution in a healthy Dutch population and in Graves' patients. An exploratory study. *Orbit*. 2004 Jan 8;23(3):161–8.

[38] Migliori ME, Gladstone GJ. Determination of the Normal Range of Exophthalmometric Values for Black and White Adults. *Am J Ophthalmol*. 1984 Oct;98(4):438–42.

[39] Vasanthakumar P, Kumar P, Rao M. Anthropometric Analysis of Palpebral Fissure Dimensions and its Position in South Indian Ethnic Adults. *Oman Med J*. 2013 Jan 16;28(1):26–32.

[40] Bhargav PRK, Sabaretnam M, Kumar SC, Zwalitha S, Devi NV. Regression of Ophthalmopathic Exophthalmos in Graves' Disease After Total Thyroidectomy: a Prospective Study of a Surgical Series. *Indian Journal of Surgery*. 2017 Dec 22;79(6):521–6.

[41] Frilling A, Goretzki PE, Grußendorf M, Erbslöh M, Röher HD. The influence of surgery on endocrine ophthalmopathy. *World J Surg*. 1990 May;14(3):442–5.

[42] Liu ZW, Masterson L, Fish B, Jani P, Chatterjee K. Thyroid surgery for Graves' disease and Graves' ophthalmopathy. Vol. 11, *Cochrane Database of Systematic Reviews*. 2015.

Chapter 10

Radioactive Iodine versus Surgery in the Management of Toxic Multinodular Goiter and Toxic Adenoma

Shawn S. Thomas[*]
and Paul M. Jacob[†]
Department of Endocrine Surgery, CMC Hospital, Vellore, Tamilnadu, India

Abstract

Toxic adenoma (TA) and toxic multinodular goiter (MNG) are treated by definitive Radioactive Iodine (RAI) therapy or surgery. The outcomes of radioactive iodine therapy depend on the size of the adenoma, uptake percentage of the nodule, and status of hyperthyroidism prior to the therapy. RAI therapy is recommended for persons who are at an increased risk of surgical complications, such as those with previous surgery or external radiation to the neck. In larger nodules > 4cms, the goiter persists despite a reduction in size after RAI.

Surgery is preferred in AFTNs, especially in the younger age group, because of the risk of malignancy in the toxic nodule, the likelihood of normal function post hemithyroidectomy, and the risk of developing malignancy in the irradiated extra-nodular thyroid tissue with RAI therapy. Definitive indications for surgery for TMNG include large goiters, suspicious features on cytology or imaging, pressure symptoms, persistent disease after ablation, and those with contraindications for RAI. Thyroidectomy has the lowest relapse rate (10%) and the highest

[*] Corresponding Author's Email: shawnthomas@cmcvellore.ac.in.
[†] Corresponding Author's Email: mjpaul@cmcvellore.ac.in.

In: Understanding and Managing Hyperthyroidism
Editor: Poongkodi Karunakaran
ISBN: 979-8-88697-636-6

cure rate (100%) as compared to the relapse rate with Anti-thyroid drugs (52%) and RAI (15%).

Keywords: radioactive iodine therapy, ablation, toxic multinodular goiter, toxic adenoma

1. Introduction

Graves' disease is the most common cause of hyperthyroidism, followed by toxic nodular goiter. Toxic nodular goiter is a clinical entity that encompasses both toxic multinodular goiter (TMNG) and toxic adenoma (TA) [1]. It accounts for 3 – 11% of cases of thyrotoxicosis and a higher percentage in iodine deficient areas. It also accounts for about 5% of cases of solitary thyroid nodules who come for evaluation [1–3]. Traditionally, these hot nodules were thought to have a significantly low risk of malignancy; hence, most guidelines did not recommend a cytological evaluation. More recent studies have, however, quoted a higher risk of malignancy and hence recommended adequate evaluation [1–4]. The teaching that hot nodules have a lower risk of malignancy stems from older studies in which scintigraphy was performed on all thyroid nodules as part of the diagnostic evaluation [5]. Sokal, in the 1950s, was probably the first to publish his report about a higher incidence of malignancy in toxic nodules compared to non-toxic nodules [6]. The risk of malignancy generally ranges from 5 – 8.2% for TMNG and 2.5 – 4.4% for TA's [7]. Co-existence of hyperthyroidism and thyroid carcinoma causes diagnostic and therapeutic dilemmas [8]. A meta-analysis and systematic review done by Lau et al., comparing 6778 nodules pooled odds ratio demonstrated a lower risk of malignancy in a toxic adenoma compared to a solitary non-toxic adenoma (OR = 0.38, 95% CI 0.25, 0.59). Similarly, the pooled odds ratio of 6658 individuals showed a lower risk of malignancy in toxic MNG as compared to non-toxic MNG (OR = 0.51, 95% CI 0.34, 0.75 and the combined pooled OR of all nodules showed a lower risk of malignancy in the toxic group as compared to the non-toxic group (OR = 0.45, 95% CI 0.31, 0.65), however the overall risk of malignancy in toxic nodules was higher than expected [5]. Giles et al., studied a cohort of 817 toxic patients; the frequency of carcinoma was 3.8% in GD, 6.4% in TMG, and 12% in TA and demonstrated a significantly higher incidence in those with cold nodules (13%) than those without cold nodules (2.9%). The malignant lesion was situated in the cold nodule in 45% of patients with cancer [7].

The treatment options for TA and TMNG include anti-thyroid drugs (ATD), radioactive iodine ablation (RAIA), or surgery.

2. Anti-Thyroid Drugs

Pharmacological agents are generally used as a bridge to definitive treatment because of the high chance of relapse when discontinued due to somatic mutation in the TSH receptors and also the risk of drug related adverse effects [1–3]. Few studies have demonstrated reduced response rates to RAIA after pre-treatment with ATD. However, there are others that do not show any effect [9, 10]. The response to RAIA is not affected by the duration of ATD's therapy before RAIA [10].

3. Radioactive Iodine Ablation

The goal of RAIA is to destroy sufficient thyroid parenchyma to make the patient either euthyroid or hypothyroid. RAIA has proven highly efficacious, especially with more than one dose. However, there is no standard regimen that assures complete remission [9]. A low fixed dose (185MBq) of radioactive iodine (RAI) results in lower rates of hypothyroidism but has risks of lower cure rates [9]. Allahabadia et al., demonstrated better response rates to 370MBq compared to 185MBq with comparable rates of hypothyroidism in both groups since low dose RAI was associated with higher relapse rates requiring further doses, which increased the rate of hypothyroidism [9]. Sake et al., demonstrated that a dose of 555MBq versus 740MBq showed a higher cure rate in the former group (100% versus 90.8%), and this they attributed to low doses being given to smaller nodules and higher success rates in smaller nodules. The cure rates in nodules < 2 cm was 100% as compared to 92% in nodules > 2 cm. They reported a comparable cure rate for both toxic MNG and toxic adenoma – 93.8% vs. 94.7% [1]. As the rest of the thyroid gland is hypo-functioning in TAs, it is less likely to accumulate RAI, and the risk of post ablative hypothyroidism is lower in this cohort [11]. Cure rates can be improved by administering higher doses to patients with adverse factors such as severe hyperthyroidism in larger volume glands. The risk of long-term hypothyroidism, irrespective of the dose of RAI administered, ranges between

2-3% every year after therapy [9]. This risk ranges from about 19% in the TMNG group to 9% in the AFTN group [10].

The outcomes following treatment of toxic nodular goiter with RAI depend on several factors, such as the size of the nodule, radioactive iodine uptake, and the level of hyperthyroidism prior to therapy. Normalization of hyperthyroidism prior to iodine therapy results in the negation of the protective effect of the toxic nodule taking up all the radioactive iodine and results in a higher incidence of hypothyroidism in treated patients [12]. Post-treatment cure rates are usually assessed at 6 months. Cure rates with RAIA range from 71 – 93.9% [1]. Response of the nodule size is variable and ranges from only a 50% reduction in the size of the nodule over 1 year to a complete resolution seen in 56.3% of treated patients [13]. Nodules > 20ml are more likely to require consequent doses of RAI to show a significant reduction in size [11]. The oncogenic effect of RAI on the thyroid gland is debatable and has not been conclusively proven [13]. The Cooperative Thyrotoxicosis Therapy Follow-up Study demonstrated a modest increase in the risk of solid cancers in patients treated with RAI for hyperthyroidism [14]. There is also evidence to suggest that the risk of death from solid cancers in patients treated for hyperthyroidism increases with a greater absorbed dose to exposed tissues, which, however, is small and observed at only higher doses. Further studies are required to confirm these findings [15]. The main advantages of RAIA are its low cost, short half-life of 8 days, and lower risk of permanent hypothyroidism.

4. Surgery

This modality has higher cure rates but is associated with a risk of hypoparathyroidism and recurrent laryngeal nerve injury [1]. In a cost-effective analysis study done by Trecan et al., which included studies from 1966 to 2001, they concluded that in women up to 72 years of age, comparing surgery, high dose RAI and ATD, surgery was most effective and least expensive compared to the others. However, in older patients with co-morbidities, if the risk of surgical morbidity was greater than 0.9%, surgery may not be the preferred strategy [3]. High-dose RAI (> 15mCi) was found to be as effective and less expensive in the age group > 65 years. The likelihood of detecting incidental thyroid cancers during surgery as per this study was 0.3 – 1.2%. However, most often these were intra-thyroidal and microscopic [3]. There are case reports of toxic nodules increasing in size following RAIA and eventually being diagnosed as cancer post-surgery because of incomplete initial evaluation, and hence the addition of FNAC before proceeding with RAIA in suspicious thyroid nodules is important [13, 16]. Surgery has the advantage of rapid control of toxicity, and permanent cure. It reduces the risk of missing thyroid malignancies which have a slightly higher propensity to be associated with solitary thyroid nodules [2]. In a retrospective review done by Vidal Trecan and others, the incidence of thyroid cancer in those undergoing thyroidectomy for toxic adenoma was 0.7% (95% CI 0.3 – 1.2%), and the adenoma rarely contained the malignancy [2]. The complications associated with surgery include transient vocal cord palsies and rarely persistent dysphonia, post-surgery hematomas, and anaesthesia related complications [2].

Another treatment option being tried at a few centers is image guided intra-lesional injection of ethanol. However, these have their own unique complications, such as pain associated with the injection, the need for multiple sessions for larger nodules, and extravasation of alcohol with the risk of injury to adjacent structures, including the recurrent laryngeal nerve [11, 17].

Conclusion

Toxic nodules that are planned for ablation should be subjected to cytological evaluation if there are any clinical or ultrasound features that appear suspicious for malignancy [18]. Surgery is a highly effective therapeutic strategy, especially in those without significant co-morbidities that could affect surgical outcomes. RAIA is a good option for elderly patients with co-morbidity. Quality of life after treatment is a significant concern especially in thyroid disorders which otherwise has a good prognosis. Patient preference should be considered while deciding on treatment options.

References

[1] Şakı H, Cengiz A, Yürekli Y. Effectiveness of Radioiodine Treatment for Toxic Nodular Goiter. *Mirt*. 2015 Oct 5;24(3):100–4.

[2] Vidal-Trecan G M, Stahl J, Durand-Zaleski I. Managing toxic thyroid adenoma: a cost-effectiveness analysis. *Eur. J. Endocrinol*. 2002 Mar 1;146(3):283–94.

[3] Vidal-Trecan G M, Stahl J E, Eckman M H. Radioiodine or Surgery for Toxic Thyroid Adenoma: Dissecting an Important Decision. A Cost-Effectiveness Analysis. *Thyroid*. 2004 Nov;14(11):933–45.

[4] Mizukami Y, Michigishi T, Nonomura A, Yokoyama K, Noguchi M, Hashimoto T, Nakamura S, Ishizaki T. Autonomously Functioning (Hot) Nodule of the Thyroid Gland: A Clinical and Histopathologic Study of 17 Cases. *Am. J. Clin. Pathol*. 1994 Jan 1;101(1):29–35.

[5] Lau L W, Ghaznavi S, Frolkis A D, Stephenson A, Robertson H L, Rabi D M, Paschke R. Malignancy risk of hyperfunctioning thyroid nodules compared with non-toxic nodules: systematic review and a meta-analysis. *Thyroid Res*. 2021 Dec;14(1):3.

[6] Sokal J E. Incidence of malignancy in toxic and nontoxic multinodular goiter. *JAMA*. 1954 Apr 17;154(16):1321.

[7] Giles (Senyurek) Y, Fatih T, Harika B, Yersu K, Tarik T, Serdar T. The risk factors for malignancy in surgically treated patients for Graves' disease, toxic multinodular goiter, and toxic adenoma. *Surgery*. 2008 Dec;144(6):1028–37.

[8] Naser I, Nagy A, Ali I, Elsebaaiae A. Value of Fine Needle Aspiration Biopsy in Toxic Thyroid Adenoma. *The Egyptian Journal Nuclear Medicine*. 2018 Dec 1;17(2):48–63.

[9] Allahabadia A, Daykin J, Sheppard M C, Gough S C L, Franklyn J A. *Radioiodine Treatment of Hyperthyroidism—Prognostic Factors for Outcome*. :7.

[10] Knapska-Kucharska M, Oszukowska L, Lewiński A. Analysis of demographic and clinical factors affecting the outcome of adioiodine therapy in patients with hyperthyroidism. *aoms*. 2010;4:611–22.

[11] Erdoğan M F, Küçük N Ö, Anl C, Aras S, Özer D, Aras G, Kamel N. Effect of radioiodine therapy on thyroid nodule size and function in patients with toxic adenomas: *Nuclear Medicine Communications*. 2004 Nov;25(11):1083–7.

[12] Ahmad T, Khoja A, Rashid N H, Ashfaq M A. Outcome of radioactive iodine therapy in Toxic Nodular Goiter in Pakistan. *Pak. J. Med. Sci*. [Internet]. 2018 Sep 7 [cited 2022 May 16];34(5). Available from: http://pjms.com.pk/index.php/pjms/article/view/15244.

[13] Uludag M, Yetkin G, Citgez B, Isgor A, Basak T. Autonomously functioning thyroid nodule treated with radioactive iodine and later diagnosed as papillary thyroid cancer. *Hormones*. 2008 Apr;7(2):175–9.

[14] Biondi B. Radioactive Iodine Treatment in Hyperthyroidism and Cancer Mortality—A Still Controversial Issue. *JAMA Netw Open*. 2021 Sep 17;4(9):e2126361.

[15] Kitahara C M, Berrington de Gonzalez A, Bouville A, Brill A B, Doody M M, Melo D R, Simon S L. Sosa J A, Tulchinsky M, Villoing D, Preston D L. Association of Radioactive Iodine Treatment With Cancer Mortality in Patients With Hyperthyroidism. *JAMA Intern. Med*. 2019 Aug 1;179(8):1034.

[16] Tfayli H M, Teot L A, Indyk J A, Witchel S F. Papillary Thyroid Carcinoma in an Autonomous Hyperfunctioning Thyroid Nodule: Case Report and Review of the Literature. *Thyroid*. 2010 Sep;20(9):1029–32.

[17] Freitas J E. Therapeutic options in the management of toxic and nontoxic nodular goiter. *Seminars in Nuclear Medicine*. 2000 Apr;30(2):88–97.

[18] Mirfakhraee S, Mathews D, Peng L, Woodruff S, Zigman J M. A solitary hyperfunctioning thyroid nodule harboring thyroid carcinoma: review of the literature. *Thyroid Res*. 2013 Dec;6(1):7.

Chapter 11

Thyroid Cancer in Graves' Disease

Tran N. Luong*
Phan H. Hiep
Nguyen G. Son†
Tran D. Ket
Pham Q. Thang
Truong Q. Huy
and Nguyen V. Hien
Thyroid Surgery Department, National Hospital of Endocrinology, Ha Noi, Vietnam

Abstract

Thyroid cancer accounts for about 1% of all cancers. The incidence of thyroid cancer is increasing worldwide, more than any other cancer. The American Thyroid Association reported a three-fold increase in thyroid cancer incidence from 4.9 per 100,000 people in 1975 to 14.3 per 100,000 people in 2009, mainly papillary thyroid carcinoma [1]. Thyroid cancer in patients with hyperthyroidism is rarely reported as a histological surprise in the thyroidectomy specimen after surgical management. But recent studies have shown an increasing incidence of thyroid cancer in hyperthyroidism, particularly in patients with Graves' disease. The reported rate of thyroid cancer in Graves' disease ranges widely up to 16,7% [2]. Graves' disease is an autoimmune disease and the most common cause of hyperthyroidism, often presenting as diffuse toxic goiter. Studies have shown that the frequency of detection of thyroid

* Corresponding Author's Email: ngocluongsurgery@yahoo.com.
† Corresponding Author's Email: sonngan82@gmail.com.

In: Understanding and Managing Hyperthyroidism
Editor: Poongkodi Karunakaran
ISBN: 979-8-88697-636-6

nodules is increased in Graves' disease and that thyroid nodules detected in Graves' disease have a higher risk of malignancy and metastatic lymph nodes compared with thyroid nodules in euthyroid patients. Hence, it is pertinent to study this clinical entity adequately. In this chapter, we will study in detail the incidence of thyroid cancer in Graves' disease and the peculiarities in the clinical manifestations, diagnosis, and management of thyroid cancer in patients with Graves' disease.

Keywords: thyroid cancer, Graves' disease, thyroid nodules

1. Introduction

The first person who described the hormonal activity of a malignant thyroid tumor was Von Eiselsberg, a German surgeon, in 1894. His patient had symptoms of myxedema caused by a mass metastasis in the sternum, which disappeared after thyroidectomy. Nevertheless, in the first decades of the twentieth century, the coexistence of thyroid cancer and hyperthyroidism was rarely reported. In 1937, Mean even stated that 'thyrotoxicosis was insurance against cancer of the thyroid.' Despite this statement, a vast number of subsequent research demonstrate that thyroid carcinoma is not unusual in patients presenting with thyrotoxicosis. Thyroid cancer associated with Graves' disease requires a distinct approach to clinical management.

Graves' disease (GD) is an autoimmune disorder of the thyroid gland. Although first described by Parry in 1825, it is best known as Graves' disease in the English-speaking world and as von Basedow's disease on the continent of Europe. This disease is considered the most common cause of hyperthyroidism. It is characterized by the presence of antibodies against thyroid peroxidase (TPO), thyroglobulin (Tg), and the TSH receptor (TSHR) in the serum [3]. The primary mechanism of GD is the activation of thyroid-stimulating autoantibodies (TSAbs), which stimulate the excess production and secretion of thyroid hormone.

On the other hand, thyroid cancer accounts for more than 95% of malignancies of the endocrine system and frequently correlates with specific genetic lesions [4]. Papillary thyroid carcinoma, the most prevalent thyroid cancer subtype, has been associated with specific genetic alterations such as BRAF mutation, RET/PTC rearrangement, TRK-T rearrangement, and RAS mutation in some recent studies. Similarly, mutations in the RAS family members (HRAS, KRAS, NRAS) are also quite common in follicular thyroid cancer (40-50%). Medullary thyroid carcinoma is associated with RET mutation. Finally, in anaplastic thyroid carcinoma, TP53 mutation is the main genetic alternation, followed by BRAF, RAS, and PIK3CA mutations [4].

Studies have shown that the frequency of detection of thyroid nodules is increased in Graves' disease and that thyroid nodules detected in Graves' disease have a higher risk of malignancy and metastatic lymph nodes compared with thyroid nodules in euthyroid patients. Hence, it is pertinent to study this clinical entity adequately. In this chapter, we will study in detail the incidence of thyroid cancer in Graves' disease and the peculiarities in the clinical manifestations, diagnosis, and management of thyroid cancer in patients with Graves' disease.

2. Epidemiology

Since the famous statement of Mean, many studies have evaluated the incidence of malignant thyroid tumors in Graves' disease patients. The rate of thyroid carcinoma found during surgery for GD is reported to vary widely, ranging up to 16.7% [2].

Table 1. Numbers of cases and rates of thyroid nodules (TN) and carcinoma (Ca) in total Graves' patients suffered from thyroidectomy in each study

Ref no	Author	Period	Total patient	GD (TN)		GD (Ca)		Rate of Ca in GD (TN) group (%)
				n	%	n	%	
[5]	Pacini	1970-1985	86	18	20.9	6	6.9	33.3
[6]	Thakur	1989-1993	49	7	14.3	4	8.2	57.1
[7]	Kraimps	1991-1997	557	140	25.1	21	3.8	15
[8]	Gerenova	1990-2000	95	46	48.4	7	7.4	15.2
[2]	Weber	1993-2005	48	12	25	8	16.7	66.7
[9]	Erbil	1996-2005	150	80	53.3	18	12	22.5
[10]	Ren	2002-2012	423	96	22.7	58	13.7	60.4
[11]	Tran Ngoc Luong	2002-2009	1163	425	36.5	24	2.1	5.6

Eight studies shown in Table 1 reported a wide prevalence of GD and thyroid cancer coexistence in various geographical regions [2, 5-11]. These retrospective studies provided data on Graves' patients who had undergone thyroid surgery (total or subtotal thyroidectomy) for many other indications. Indications for surgery included failure and adverse effects of anti-thyroid drugs or the appearance of suspicious malignant nodules. The proportion of thyroid nodules in Graves' patients fluctuates from 8% to 53.3%, whereas the prevalence of cancer concurrent with GD ranges from 2.1% to 16.7%. Cancer occurs in a group of GD (TN) with an even higher frequency, from 5.6% to 66.7%. According to the American thyroid association, the prevalence of palpable thyroid nodules is about 5% in females and 1% in men living in iodine-sufficient parts of the world. It can even be up to 68% detected by ultrasonography (US) in a group of randomly selected individuals, while thyroid cancer appears in 7-15% of cases depending on age, sex, radiation exposure history, family history, and other factors [1]. It seems similar to the prevalence found in epidemiological studies when sonography was used to examine thyroid morphology, but the incidence rate of thyroid cancer in GD is higher than the overall population figures. These studies show that the risk of malignancy increases significantly in Graves' patients with thyroid cancer.'

The National Health and Nutrition Examination Survey (NHANES III) data from the United States showed the female preponderance of thyroid disease including thyroid cancer and GD. The result has indicated a men-to-women ratio of approximately one-tenth in GD. Several studies showed a similar proportion of male to female ratio in GD patients with thyroid cancer, and female patients accounted for 60% to 87% of the cases.

3. Pathogenesis

The relationship between thyroid cancer and GD is still unclear, but several recent studies have put forth some hypotheses. The central mechanism of GD is the occurrence of autoantibodies directed against the TSH receptor (TSHRAbs), which behave as thyroid-stimulating antibodies. These antibodies compete with the binding of TSH to its specific receptor site in the cell membrane and can activate adenyl cyclase. Thyroid neoplastic cells also have functional receptors for TSH, so Belfiore 1989 reported the ability of TSHRAbs to stimulate the growth and function of neoplastic thyroid cells in patients with concurrent GD.

In autoimmune thyroid diseases, T cells are reactive to thyroid antigens and peptides derived from these antigens. Intrathyroidal T cells from patients with GD include helper T- cell subtype 1 (Th1) (which secrets interleukin-2 (IL2) and interferon ɣ) and helper T- cell subtype 2 (Th2) (which secrets interleukin-4 (IL4)). The predominant active T lymphocyte is the Th2 subset, and the level of IL4 in the serum of Graves' patients was markedly elevated. IL4 is a pleiotropic cytokine that elicits the main impact on the immune response by causing proliferation and apoptosis inhibition in both B and T cells. Moreover, it also induces IgE and IgG1 class switching and major histocompatibility complex class II molecule expression [12]. Recently, IL4 receptors (IL-4Rα) were found in cells from various epithelial malignant tumors such as thyroid, renal, colon, and breast cancer. Veronica Vella et al. demonstrated the invivo relevance of IL-4 in thyroid cancer [13]. It may increase the viability of malignant cells by potentiating the role of other antiapoptotic factors such as IGFs. An impaired ability of the cell to undergo apoptosis in response to genotoxic insults causes the gathering of mutations that may result in malignant transformation. This phenomenon explains the increasing rate of thyroid cancer in GD patients. In addition, IL4 also stimulates chemoinvasion, making thyroid cancer cells more aggressive and allowing hematogenous dissemination. Many studies showed a markedly higher incidence of distant metastases and recurrence of thyroid cancer in GD patients compared with similar tumors appearing in euthyroid patients.

4. Clinical Symptoms

Patients with the coexistence of thyroid cancer and Graves' disease have a clinical picture of both diseases. The classic features of Graves' disease include diffuse goiter, thyrotoxicosis, infiltrative orbitopathy, and sporadic infiltrative dermopathy. However, the appearance of malignant thyroid tumors in GD patients makes some differences in the thyroid gland. In most Graves' disease patients, the thyroid gland is symmetrically enlarged and has consistency varying from soft to firm and rubbery. On the other hand, in Graves' patients with concomitant thyroid cancer, the thyroid gland frequently has an asymmetrical shape and firm consistency depending on the size of the tumors. In addition, the metastasis to lymph nodes in the neck may be hard and palpable to patients or physicians. Recently, with the widespread use of high-frequency neck ultrasound for the evaluation of GD patients, most thyroid cancers may be detected at an early stage, even before the manifestation of thyroid carcinoma symptoms. The presentation of thyrotoxicosis, orbitopathy, and dermopathy in GD patients with concurrent thyroid cancer is similar to normal GD patients.

Clinical manifestations of thyrotoxicosis or hyperthyroidism involve almost any organ system such as cardiovascular, nervous, alimentary, skeletal, hematopoietic system, muscle, skin, hair, protein, carbohydrate, and lipid metabolism. Patients frequently report nervousness, irritability, easy fatigability, inability to concentrate, and intolerance to heat. There is often significant weight loss in spite of increased appetite. Other common symptoms are excessive sweating, mild or moderate muscle weakness, and hand tremors. In patients over 60 years of age, cardiovascular and myopathic symptoms may predominate with the most common presenting complaints of palpitation, tachycardia, dyspnea on exertion, tremor, weight loss, and nervousness. In addition, atrial fibrillation, splenomegaly, and gynecomastia can occur.

Graves' ophthalmopathy appears in 40-60% of patients. Hyperthyroidism may occur several years before presenting any eye symptoms in 30% of cases, and only in approximately 10% of patients may the eye manifestation precede the thyroidal symptoms [14]. Clinical signs are lid retraction, edema, exophthalmos, motility disorders, and visual impairments. The American Thyroid Association (ATA) has classified the eye symptoms in GD by inducing a mnemonic system in which the first letters of each category constitute the term NOSPECS.

Dermopathy is relatively rare, occurring in less than 5% of patients with GD, and is almost always accompanied by GO with a high serum titer of TSH receptor antibodies. It is described as the thickening of the skin, particularly over the pretibial area, due to the accumulation of glycosaminoglycans.

5. Laboratory Tests

The laboratory findings in GD are essentially the combination of a suppressed serum TSH level and elevated serum T3 and T4 levels. Thyroid cancer rarely affects serum TSH levels. Measuring thyrotropin receptor autoantibodies may be helpful to indicate the degree of disease in an individual GD patient. Demonstration of TSHRAbs may also be of diagnostic value in the euthyroid patient with exophthalmos. Additionally, TSHRAb testing is useful in the prognostication of GD patients who are treated with antithyroid drugs. Several studies reported that a permanently high level of TSHRAbs is an important predictor of recurrence on cessation of the drug [15].

Thyroglobulin (Tg) is a thyroid-specific glycoprotein that serves as the source of thyroid hormone production within the lumen of thyroid follicles. The amount of Tg may be increasingly released into the bloodstream in follicular thyroid cancer (FTC). Unfortunately, there is an overlap of serum Tg levels in FTC and several benign thyroid diseases, so the measurement of serum Tg levels is not useful in diagnosing a thyroid nodule. In addition, increased calcitonin level may be specific for medullary thyroid cancer

(MTC), but the rarity of MTC makes the routine measurement of calcitonin not always necessary.

Ultrasonography is a noninvasive technique and becoming an essential part of clinical examination. Sonography may provide adequate information for physicians, including the shape, size, and lesion in thyroid parenchyma. Thyroid nodules even smaller than 5mm in diameter can be readily detected. Recently, the American College of Radiology (ACR) published the Thyroid Imaging, Reporting and Data System (TIRADS) which has been widely accepted in many countries [16]. ACR TIRADS is based on five categories to assess thyroid tumors including composition, echogenicity, shape, margin, and echogenic foci as below:

Composition (Choose 1)	Echogenicity (Choose 1)	Shape (Choose 1)	Margin (Choose 1)	Echogenic Foci (Choose 1)
+Cystic or almost completely cystic **0 points** + Spongform **0 points** + Mixed cystic and solid **1 points** + Solid or almost completely solid **2 point**	+ Anechoic **0 points** + Hyperechoic or isoechoic **1 points** + Hypoechoic **2 points** + Very hypoechoic **3 points**	+Wider-than- tall **0 points** Taller-than-wide **3 points**	+ Smooth **0 points** + Ill- difined **0 points** + Lobulated or irregular **2 points** + Extra – thyroidal extension **3 points**	+ None or large comet – tail artifacts **0 points** + Macrocacifications **1 points** + Peripheral (rim) calcifications **2 points** + Punctate echogenic **3 points**

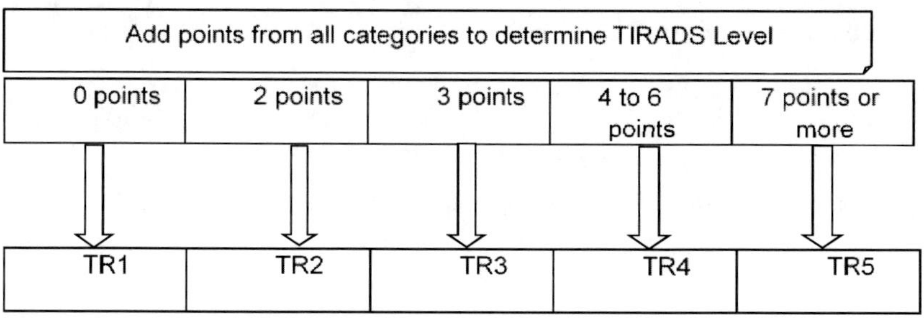

Figure 1. Chart showing five categories on the basis of the ACR Thyroid Imaging, Reporting and Data System (TI-RADS) lexicon, TR levels, and criteria for fine-needle aspiration or follow-up ultrasound. Explanatory notes appear at the bottom [16].

The point total determines the nodule's ACR TI-RADS level, which ranges from TR1 (benign) to TR5 (high suspicion of malignancy). This classification is useful in the diagnosis cancer capability of thyroid tumors. In patient with known thyroid cancer, sonography can be functional in evaluating the extent of disease. It also provides information about any sonographically suspicious regional lymph nodes and thereby surgeons can permit planning of the extent of nodal dissection. Furthermore, post-thyroidectomy observation need sonography to detect residual, recurrent or metastasis disease in the neck.

In patients with coexistence of thyroid nodules and GD, thyroid scintigraphy plays an integral part in excluding a toxic adenoma or toxic multinodular goiter. Radionuclide scanning uses technetium-99 pertechnetate (^{99m}Tc) or radioactive iodine ^{123}I. Radioisotope scanning allows further assessment of thyroid-functional anatomy. Basically, radioisotope scanning divides image of thyroid tumor into hypofunctioning (cold), isofunctioning (warm) and hyperfunctioning (hot) nodule. Most thyroid cancers are inefficient in trapping and organifying iodine and occur on scans as cold nodules. Unfortunately, most benign thyroid tumors also do not accumulate iodine and thereby are cold nodules. Approximately 1–20% of cold nodules are malignant, as compared with less than 4% of hot nodules [17].

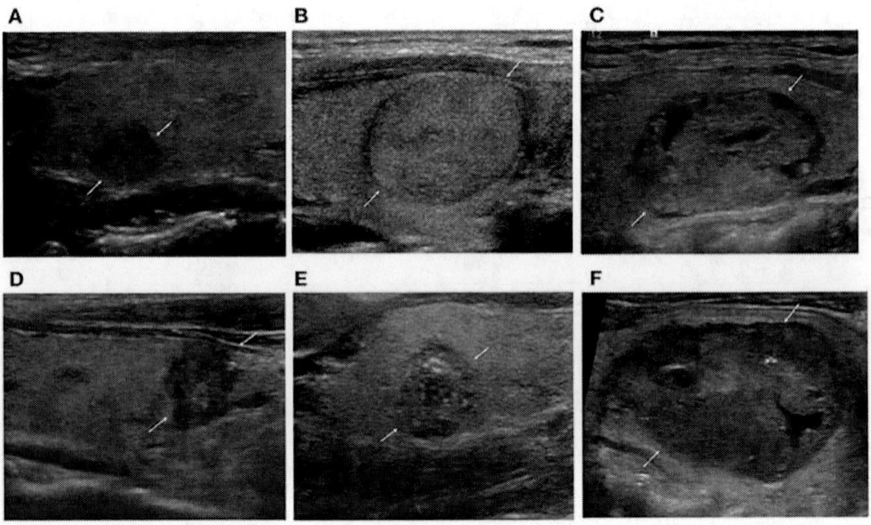

Figure 2. (A) Nodular goiter. Solid and hypoechoic nodule. ACR-TIRADS. (B) Follicular adenoma. Solid and isoechoic nodule. ACR-TIRADS, 3 (C) Follicular adenoma. Mixed cystic and solid. ACR-TIRADS, 3. (D) Papillary thyroid carcinoma. Solid and hypoechoic nodule with taller-than-wide shape, irregular margins, and microcalcification. ACR-TIRADS, 5 (E) Papillary thyroid carcinoma. Solid and hypoechoic nodule with microcalcification and macrocalcification. ACR-TIRADS, 5. (F) Medullary thyroid carcinoma. Mostly solid and hypoechoic nodule with dispersed microcalcifications. ACR-TIRADS, 5.

Table 2. The Bethesda System for Reporting Thyroid Cytopathology: Diagnostic Categories and Risk of Malignancy

Category	Risk of malignancy in 2009 Bethesda system	Risk of malignancy in 2017 Bethesda system
I. Nondiagnostic or'' unsatisfactory	1-4	5-10
II. Benign	0-3	0-3
III. Atypia of'' undetermined significance or follicular lesion of undetermined significance	5-15	10-30
IV. Follicular neoplasm or suspicious follicular neoplasm	15-30	25-40
V. Suspicious for malignancy	60-75	50-75
VI. Malignancy	97-99	97-99

Fine needle aspiration biopsy (FNAB) of thyroid nodules plays the most important role in the diagnosis of thyroid cancer. It is reported overall rates of sensitivity and specificity exceeding 90% in iodine-sufficient geographical areas. In severe hyperthyroidism, the risk of thyroid storm following thyroid surgery or other manipulation had been recorded in the literature. So that, in Graves' patients with thyroid cancer, FNAB should be performed if patients achieve euthyroid status.'

Recently, ATA recommended that the thyroid nodules FNA cytology should be reported using diagnostic group outlined in the Bethesda System for Reporting Thyroid Cytopathology [1]. It has been adopted widely in United States and in many centers worldwide. It was published for the first time in 2009 and then, was updated in 2017. The Bethesda system recognizes six diagnostic categories including: (I) Nondiagnostic or unsatisfactory, (II) Benign, (III) Atypia of undetermined significance or follicular lesion of undetermined significance, (IV) Follicular neoplasm or suspicious follicular neoplasm, (V) Suspicious for malignancy, (VI) Malignancy.

Each category has an implied malignant cancer that's varies from 0-3% for benign category to 97-99% for malignancy category. After many studies, the features for category I, II, IV and V are updated in the 2017 revision with the increased data in these diagnostic categories. This flexible framework has facilitated communication among cytopathologists, endocrinologists, surgeons, radiologists, and other health care providers; facilitate cytologic-histologic correlation for thyroid diseases; facilitate research into the epidemiology, molecular biology, pathology, and diagnosis of thyroid diseases; and allow easy and reliable sharing of data from different laboratories for national and international collaborative studies.

6. Treatment

According to ATA, if Graves' disease patient harbor thyroid nodules with cytopathology suspicious or diagnostic of malignancy, surgery may be considered the best choice. This recommendation is agreed by many authors because of some significant advantages of surgery over I131 including rapid control of hyperthyroidism, immediate relief of pressure symptoms in patients with large volume goiter and decreased recurrent rates of both Graves' disease and thyroid cancer. Subtotal thyroidectomy for Graves' disease is associated with a high rate of recurrence [18] and maybe not the optimal treatment approach. Hence, total thyroidectomy is now well established as the procedure of surgery in Graves' patients with concurrent thyroid carcinoma. However, there has been a controversy surrounding the proper extent of surgery for those patients. In the past, some surgeons suggested radical surgery involving at least total thyroidectomy and lymph node dissection followed by radioiodine treatment. On the other hand, the present studies indicate that the procedure of choice should depend on the diagnostic timing and stage of the tumor. These authors suggest that the extent of surgery should be similar to thyroid cancer in euthyroid cancer. In differentiated thyroid cancer, National Comprehensive Cancer Network (NCCN) guidelines suggest therapeutic neck dissection of the involved compartment for clinical apparent/ biopsy-proven disease, and routine prophylactic central neck dissection is not indicated in most papillary thyroid cancers.

Thyroid surgery for patients with Graves' disease is generally more difficult and technically challenging than for normal patients with thyroid nodules because of the increased vascularity of the thyroid gland. It is a high risk surgery that can cause heavy intraoperative bleeding. However, surgery for patients with coexisting thyroid cancer and GD is even more complex than Graves' disease alone due to the invasion into critically important adjacent structures and metastatic nature of the malignant cells. So that, to reduce the risk of complications, preparation for surgery become significantly important. Antithyroid agents may decrease the morbidity and mortality rates of surgery for Graves' disease because these drugs deplete glandular hormone stores and restore the euthyroid status. Nevertheless, these drugs do not impair the hypervascularity of thyroid gland in short-term unless TSHRAb level reduces. On the other hand, iodine may cause a decrease in height of follicular cells, enlargement of follicles with retention of colloid and reduction of hypervascularity. Often, after the metabolic state is restore to normal, oral Lugol's' solution (potassium iodide, SSKI) is administered preoperatively (2 to 3 drops twice daily) for a further 7 to 10 days. During this period, the thyroid gland may become firm and smaller, so that, postoperative complications can be reduced to minimum. Finally, surgery for Graves' patients with concurrent thyroid carcinomas need to be performed by experienced surgeons in the high-volume centers.

Because the hazards after thyroid surgery depend on skill and experience of the surgical team, it is impossible to generalize about the frequency of complications. Major complications of total thyroidectomy include vocal cord paralysis secondary to recurrent laryngeal nerve injury and hypocalcemia due to resection of parathyroid glands. In addition, bleeding into the operative site is also a serious postoperative complication which may rapidly produce death by asphyxia. It is caused by the carelessness of surgeons in controlling intraoperative blood vessel such as the superior and/or inferior thyroid artery. This complication requires immediate evacuation of the blood and ligation of the bleeding vessel. The incidences of these complications following total thyroidectomy were reported in many studies (Table 3).

Table 3. Incidence of postoperative complication

	n	RLN paralysis		Hypocalcemia		Compressive hematoma
		Transient	Permanent	Transient	Permanent	
Thomusch (2000) [19]	7266	2.1	1.1	6.4	1.5	2.7
Rosato (2004) [20]	9599	2.4	1.3	14	2.2	1.6
Efremidou (2009) [21]	932	0.2	1.3	7.3	0.3	0.2
Duclos (2012) [22]	3574	0	2.08	20.05	2.69	0

These data are drawn from the largest published studies and reflect the rate of complications seen at centers of expertise [19-22]. The prevalence of these complications vary but it was reported to be higher in patient with Graves' disease and thyroid cancer.

To decrease the risk of RLN paralysis, the recurrent nerve should be identified systematically in every cases. Recently, neural monitoring has been used widely in many centers which was developed to help surgeons identify intraoperatively the nerve, and the it may limit this postoperative complication [23]. In a comparison of RLN identification by classical dissection versus neural monitoring (NM) in a series of 1000 cases suffer from total thyroidectomy, the result indicated that the NM diminished the prevalence of transient RLN paresis [23]. The unilateral RLN injury often causes dysphonia that usually decreases in a few weeks but that may leave the patient slightly hoarse. The bilateral vocal cord in adduction presents as acute dyspnea and is the evident at the time of extubation, requiring urgent airway re-intubation. This is a life-threatening complication and hence, thyroidectomy for the Graves' patient with thyroid cancer should be performed by high-volume surgeons only.'

Hypoparathyroidism can be either transient or permanent. The prevalence of postoperative hypocalcemia varies depending on the experiment of surgeons (Table 3). Hypoparathyroidism results from inadvertent removal of some parathyroid glands which impaired secretion of parathyroid hormones (PTH). This fact usually results in hypocalcemia associated with hyperphosphatemia. The earliest symptom of hypoparathyroidism may be anxiety and mental depression, followed by paresthesia and heightened neuromuscular excitability, such as Chvostek's and Trousseau's signs and carpopedal spasm. The PTH level is often low and sometimes undetectable. The calcium level is subnormal and the inorganic phosphate level is often increased. The severe hypoparathyroidism should be treated urgently with intravenous calcium gluconate. If patients have milder symptoms, treatment consists of daily administration of calcium and vitamin D. Doses should be adapted based on weekly measurement of calcium and phosphate levels until biological equilibrium is achieved.

Another complication should be mentioned is chyle leak caused by thoracic duct injury when thyroid surgery is combined with lymph node dissection. This is a rare but serious complication that occurs in 0.5-1.4% [24] of thyroidectomies and 2-8% of neck dissections [23-24]. If chyle leak is identified intraoperatively, the thoracic duct injury should be ligated immediately. However, ligation is not easy because identification of the duct is often difficult. In such cases, suturing the surrounding middle or deep cervical fascia over the duct leak may be possible. Some surgeons suggest to use the clavicular head of the sternocleidomastoid muscle, because it may be more bulky and there is less risk of damaging the phrenic nerve [25]. Recently, some topical agents could be used to reinforce the successful suture ligation such as cyanoacrylate adhesives, fibrin glue and polyglactin (Vicryl) mesh with encouraging results. If the chyle leak is diagnosed postoperatively, treatment approach depends on drain output, patient comorbidities, available institutional expertise and surgeon preference. Chyle leak may be categorized as low output (<500ml/ day) or high output (>500ml/ day). In general, low output chyle leak may be treated conservatively and high output chyle leak need surgical intervention to ligate the duct injury which is not recognized intraoperatively [26]. The conservative treatment includes dietary measures such as an elemental diet with medium chain triglycerides or by total parenteral nutrition and somatostatin or octreotide [27].

After total thyroidectomy, followed by iodine-131 (^{131}I) ablation of thyroid remnants, for differentiated thyroid cancer (DTC), the follow up protocol is: if no uptake is seen outside the thyroid bed on the total body scan (TBS) performed after 4-7 days after the administration of ^{131}I to destroy the thyroid remnant, T4 treatment is initiated. Many studies confirmed that ^{131}I treatment ablates only residual micro/macroscopic tumor cells in the thyroid and/or distant metastasis but does not affect healthy tissues in the body. When the Tg level obtained after withdrawal of thyroid hormone treatment is above some arbitrary limit (i.e., 10 ng/mL in our hospital), even in the absence of any other evidence of disease, 3.7 GBq (100 mCi) of ^{131}I are administered with a TBS performed 4–7 days later; this will detect radiotracer uptake outside the thyroid bed in 60–80% of patients.

7. Prognosis

Although all histological types of thyroid cancer have been found in patients with Graves' disease, many studies indicated that papillary carcinoma histology is the exclusive subtype [14, 18]. It is similar to the histological feature of thyroid cancer in the euthyroid group. In 1990, Belfiore reported the increased aggressiveness of thyroid carcinoma in Graves' patients which has been accepted widely until the next decade. The cumulative risk for recurrent/progressive distant metastases was about 3-folds higher in patients with GD than in patients in control group. After a follow-up period ranging from 50 to 363 months, approximately 30% of patients with GD had died of cancer, whereas this proportion in the control group was only 3% [13-14]. After that, this opinion had been reinforced by some studies which reported the important role of TSHRAb and IL4 (mentioned in pathogenesis). However, recent studies show that the difference between the disease-free survival and distant metastasis during the follow-up period of the patient with Graves' disease and euthyroid patient with thyroid cancer is not significant. The reason for these discordant results is the differences in criteria in the preoperative selection of patients, in the thyroid pathologic examination and in the surgical and postsurgical management of the patient. Belfiore' study was performed during period from 1982 to 1994 while ultrasound was not used widely in observation for Graves' disease. Therefore, the tumor stage is more advanced in this study compared to recent studies. In recent studies, there is a large portion of microcarcinoma (tumor's diameter <1cm), so that the metastasis rate is very low in both groups and the time of follow-up is often 5 years which is too short to observe cancer related mortality for small thyroid cancer. In addition, the differences in environmental and genetic factors between cohorts of these studies also may have influenced the varying results. Moreover, in Belfiore's study, occult cancers were excluded which might include thyroid nodules with uncertain malignant potential and have an excellent prognosis.

In 2020, Kwon demonstrated that GD is not associated with recurrence (HR 1.12, 95% CI 0.15-8.34) whereas tumor size (HR 1.58, 95% CI 1.24-2.01) and lymph node metastasis (HR 2.48. 95% CI 1.09-5.66) is the predictive factors for recurrence. A recent meta-analysis indicated that tumor size over 2cm (OR 2.69, 95% CI 2.06-3.5) and the presence of cervical lymph node metastases (OR 3.24, 95% CI 2.61- 4.02) significantly increased the rate of recurrence. Medals and colleagues also agreed with this point in their study in 2019 [28].

Conclusion

Thyroid cancer is relatively frequent in Graves' disease patients with the rate ranging up to 16.7%. In late stage, the malignant tumors in GD patients may be more aggressive than thyroid cancer occurring in matched euthyroid patients and cause higher cancer-specific mortality. However, microcarcinoma in GD does not show more aggressive behavior than in the euthyroid control group. We suggest that Graves' disease patients should undergo a detailed thyroid gland examination by routine ultrasound to identify the tumor in the early stage. Total thyroidectomy followed by I^{131} may be the optimal treatment approach for the coexistence of GD and thyroid cancer and the choice of extent of surgery should depend on the staging at the time of diagnosis and factors predicting recurrences such as lymph node metastasis and tumor size over 1 cm. Given the high risk and difficulty of this procedure, we recommend that the surgery should be performed by an experienced surgeon in a high-volume center.

References

[1] Haugen BR, Alexander EK, Bible KC, 2015 American Thyroid Association Management Guidelines for Adult Patients with Thyroid Nodules and Differentiated

Thyroid Cancer: The American Thyroid Association Guidelines Task Force on Thyroid Nodules and Differentiated Thyroid Cancer. *Thyroid Off J Am Thyroid Assoc*. 2016 Jan;26 (1):1–133.

[2] Weber KJ, Solorzano CC, Lee JK, Thyroidectomy remains an effective treatment option for Graves' disease. *Am J Surg*. 2006 Mar;191 (3):400–5.

[3] Smith TJ, Hegedüs. Graves' Disease. *N Engl J Med*. 2016 Oct 20;375 (16):1552–65.

[4] M Santoro, T J Fahey, molecular pathogenesis of thyroid neoplasia. In: *Surgery of thyroid and parathyroid gland.* Second. Philadelphia: Elsevier Saunders; 2012. p. 167–73.

[5] Pacini F, Elisei R, Di Coscio GC. Thyroid carcinoma in thyrotoxic patients treated by surgery. *J Endocrinol Invest*. 1988 Feb 1;11 (2):107–12.

[6] Thakur S, Sharma AK, Agarwal A. Carcinoma in Graves' disease. *J Assoc Physicians India*. 1995 Sep;43 (9):600–1.

[7] Kraimps J, Bouin-Pineau M, Mathonnet M, De Calan L, Multicentre study of thyroid nodules in patients with Graves' disease. *Br J Surg*. 2000 Aug;87 (8):1111–3.

[8] Gerenova J, Buysschaert M, de Burbure CY, Daumerie C. Prevalence of thyroid cancer in Graves' disease: a retrospective study of a cohort of 103 patients treated surgically. *Eur J Intern Med*. 2003 Aug;14 (5):321–5.

[9] Erbil Y, Barbaros U, Özbey N, Kapran Y, Tükenmez M, Bozbora A, Graves' disease, with and without nodules, and the risk of thyroid carcinoma. *J Laryngol Otol*. 2007/08/15 ed. 2008;122 (3):291–5.

[10] Ren M, Wu MC, Shang CZ. Predictive Factors of Thyroid Cancer in Patients with Graves' Disease. *World J Surg*. 2014 Jan 1;38 (1):80–7.

[11] Tran Ngoc Luong. Thyroid cancer and concurrent Graves' disease. *Viet Namese Journal of military medicine*. 2011;253–8.

[12] Nelms K, Keegan AD, Zamorano J, The IL-4 receptor: signaling mechanisms and biologic functions. *Annu Rev Immunol*. 1999; 17:701–38.

[13] Vella V, Mineo R, Frasca. Interleukin-4 Stimulates Papillary Thyroid Cancer Cell Survival: Implications in Patients with Thyroid Cancer and Concomitant Graves' Disease. *J Clin Endocrinol Metab*. 2004 Jun 1;89 (6):2880–9.

[14] Bartley GB, Fatourechi V, Kadrmas EF, Jacobsen SJ, The Chronology of Graves' Ophthalmopathy in an Incidence Cohort. *Am J Ophthalmol*. 1996 Apr 1;121 (4):426–34.

[15] Stöhr M, Oeverhaus M, Lytton SD. Predicting the Relapse of Hyperthyroidism in Treated Graves' Disease with Orbitopathy by Serial Measurements of TSH-Receptor Autoantibodies. *Horm Metab Res Horm Stoffwechselforschung Horm Metab*. 2021 Apr;53 (4):235–44.

[16] Tessler FN, Middleton WD, Grant EG, Hoang JK. ACR Thyroid Imaging, Reporting and Data System (TI-RADS): White Paper of the ACR TI-RADS Committee. *J Am Coll Radiol JACR*. 2017 May;14 (5):587–95.

[17] Ashcraft MW, Van Herle AJ. Management of thyroid nodules. I: History and physical examination, blood tests, X-ray tests, and ultrasonography. *Head Neck Surg*. 1981 Feb;3 (3):216–30.

[18] Wilhelm SM, McHenry CR. Total thyroidectomy is superior to subtotal thyroidectomy for management of Graves' disease in the United States. *World J Surg*. 2010 Jun;34 (6):1261–4.

[19] Thomusch O, Machens A, Sekulla C. Multivariate Analysis of Risk Factors for Postoperative Complications in Benign Goiter Surgery: Prospective Multicenter Study in Germany. *World J Surg*. 2000 Nov 1;24 (11):1335–41.

[20] Rosato L, Avenia N, Bernante P. Complications of thyroid surgery: analysis of a multicentric study on 14,934 patients operated on in Italy over 5 years. *World J Surg*. 2004 Mar;28 (3):271–6.

[21] Efremidou EI, Papageorgiou MS, Liratzopoulos N. The efficacy and safety of total thyroidectomy in the management of benign thyroid disease: a review of 932 cases. *Can J Surg J Can Chir*. 2009 Feb;52 (1):39–44.

[22] Duclos A, Peix J-L, Colin C. Influence of experience on performance of individual surgeons in thyroid surgery: prospective cross sectional multicentre study. *BMJ*. 2012 Jan 10;344:d8041.

[23] Chiang F-Y, Lee K-W, Chen H-C. Standardization of Intraoperative Neuromonitoring of Recurrent Laryngeal Nerve in Thyroid Operation. *World J Surg*. 2010 Feb 1;34 (2):223–9.

[24] Rammal A, Zawawi F, Varshney R. Chyle leak: A rare complication post-hemithyroidectomy. Case report and review of literature. *Otolaryngol Pol*. 2014 Jul 1;68 (4):204–7.

[25] Ilczyszyn A, Ridha H, Durrani AJ. Management of chyle leak post neck dissection: a case report and literature review. *J Plast Reconstr Aesthetic Surg JPRAS*. 2011 Sep;64 (9):e223-230.

[26] Delaney SW, Shi H, Shokrani A. Management of Chyle Leak after Head and Neck Surgery: Review of Current Treatment Strategies. Betka J, editor. *Int J Otolaryngol*. 2017 Jan 19;2017:8362874.

[27] Jain A, Singh SN, Singhal P. A prospective study on the role of octreotide in management of chyle fistula neck. *The Laryngoscope*. 2015 Jul;125 (7):1624–7.

[28] Medas F, Canu GL, Boi F. Predictive Factors of Recurrence in Patients with Differentiated Thyroid Carcinoma: A Retrospective Analysis on 579 Patients. *Cancers*. 2019 Aug 22;11 (9).

Chapter 12

The Management of Hyperthyroidism during Pregnancy

Kripa Elizabeth Cherian and Thomas V. Paul*

Department of Endocrinology, Christian Medical College and Hospital, Vellore, India

Abstract

The diagnosis of hyperthyroidism may be challenging in pregnancy as there is considerable overlap in the symptoms of pregnancy and hyperthyroidism. Moreover, the physiological changes associated with pregnancy could alter thyroid function tests. Gestational transient thyrotoxicosis and Graves' disease are the most common causes of hyperthyroidism in pregnancy. While gestational transient thyrotoxicosis is usually self-limiting and does not require specific treatment, antithyroid drugs are the mainstay of therapy for Graves' disease during pregnancy. Graves' disease in pregnancy warrants careful fetal surveillance through serial ultrasound monitoring for the development of adverse effects. As hyperthyroidism in pregnancy may adversely affect both maternal and fetal outcomes, early recognition and optimum management of the same are warranted.

Keywords: gestational hyperthyroidism, pregnancy, gestational transient hyperthyroidism

---

* Corresponding Author's Email: thomasvpaul@yahoo.com.

In: Understanding and Managing Hyperthyroidism
Editor: Poongkodi Karunakaran
ISBN: 979-8-88697-636-6

1. Introduction

Hyperthyroidism refers to an excess of circulating thyroid hormones in the blood due to a hyperfunction of the thyroid gland. As the clinical manifestations of hyperthyroidism may overlap with the pregnant state itself, this may pose a challenge to diagnosis. Moreover, uncontrolled hyperthyroidism in pregnancy may adversely affect the pregnant mother and the developing fetus. Thus, early recognition and appropriate treatment of hyperthyroidism are crucial to ensure adequate maternal and fetal well-being during pregnancy [1].

1.1. Epidemiology

Although thyroid disease is common during pregnancy, hyperthyroidism is less common and occurs in about 1-2% of pregnancies [2]. Gestational transient hyperthyroidism and Graves' disease (GD) are the most common causes of hyperthyroidism in pregnancy. Gestational transient hyperthyroidism is more common than GD and occurs in the first half of pregnancy in about 1-3% of pregnancies, with higher frequency noted in hyperemesis gravidarum, multiple gestations, and trophoblastic disease due to marked elevation of hCG [3].

1.2. Physiology of Thyroid Function in Pregnancy

During pregnancy, the levels of placental human chorionic glycoprotein (hCG), a 37 kDa, increase and reach their maximum by 8-11 weeks of gestation [4]. As it is structurally similar to the thyroid stimulating hormone (TSH), it acts on the maternal TSH receptors on the thyroid gland stimulating it to increase total thyroxine secretion, resulting in a transient increase in free thyroxine levels and a consequent suppression of TSH [5].

Moreover, there is an estrogen stimulated increase in levels of thyroxine binding globulin (TBG) which peaks a few weeks after conception and plateaus by mid-gestation [6]. The mechanism of this increase is attributed to the increased rate of synthesis by the liver and decreased clearance of the protein from the plasma [7]. This increase in TBG leads to higher binding of total thyroxine, a mild decrease in the concentration of free thyroxine, and a consequent rise in TSH, which is manifest in the second trimester of pregnancy [8].

In early gestation, placental deiodinase 2 ensures increased conversion of tetra-iodothyronine (T4) to tri-iodothyronine (T3), and this is responsible for maintaining adequate intra-placental T3 for trophoblast development and differentiation. Placental deiodinase 3, on the other hand, increases the conversion of T4 to rT3 (reverse T3) and T3 to di-iodothyronine (T2). As this prevents activation of T4 and inactivates T3, the fetus is protected from excess maternal thyroid hormones in the background of an increased maternal hormone demand [9].

Also, during pregnancy, there is a reduction in the total maternal iodide pool owing to an increased production of thyroid hormones, with increased renal clearance and enhanced transfer to the growing fetus. Thus, in toto, the various physiological changes that occur during pregnancy are meant to ensure the best pregnancy outcome and promote normal development of the fetus [9].

1.3. Overt versus Subclinical Hyperthyroidism

Hyperthyroidism in pregnancy may be classified biochemically as overt or subclinical. Overt hyperthyroidism refers to suppressed TSH below the pregnancy-specific reference range (<0.1mIU/L) with high total or free T3/T4 for the pregnancy specific reference range [10]. Subclinical hyperthyroidism refers to suppressed TSH with normal total or free T3/T4 for pregnancy specific reference range. Total T3/T4 values in pregnancy are 1.5 times the non-pregnancy reference range [10].

1.4. Causes of Thyrotoxicosis in Pregnancy

Excess thyroid hormone production in pregnancy may be due to multiple causes as follows [11]:

(a) *Excessive TSH-receptor stimulation* due to Graves' disease (TSH-receptor autoantibodies), gestational transient thyrotoxicosis (hCG induced), trophoblastic disease, and TSH producing pituitary adenoma
(b) *Autonomous thyroid hormone secretion* due to a toxic multi-nodular goiter, solitary toxic adenoma, activating TSH receptor mutation

(c) *Extra-thyroidal source of thyroid hormones* due to struma ovarii and functional thyroid cancer metastases

Subacute painful or painless thyroiditis with passive thyroid hormone release from a damaged thyroid gland are among the uncommon causes of thyrotoxicosis in pregnancy, while other conditions such as a TSH-secreting pituitary adenoma, struma ovarii, functional thyroid cancer metastases, or germline TSH receptor mutations are very rare.

1.5. Clinical Features and Consequences of Hyperthyroidism in Pregnancy

Clinical manifestations of hyperthyroidism may mimic some of the symptoms encountered in normal pregnancy and include palpitations, tremors, heat intolerance, and excess sweating. However, the presence of a goiter, thyroid associated ophthalmopathy, features suggesting congestive cardiac failure, inappropriate weight loss, and excessive anxiety should prompt testing for hyperthyroidism [12].

The specific features of goiter and thyroid eye disease suggest a diagnosis of GD. In the absence of a prior history of thyroid disease, with no stigmata of GD (goiter, thyroid eye disease), the presence of a self-limited mild disorder and symptoms of emesis favor the diagnosis of gestational transient hyperthyroidism [13]. The presence of severe nausea and vomiting may also be encountered in a gestational trophoblastic disease and molar pregnancy, which could be excluded by an ultrasound scan of the abdomen [14].

Mild hyperthyroidism is generally well tolerated in pregnancy and usually does not have adverse outcomes. Uncontrolled moderate to severe hyperthyroidism may be detrimental and lead to spontaneous abortions, premature delivery, low birth weight, stillbirth, eclampsia, and heart failure. The state of pregnancy can rarely precipitate a thyroid storm during labor [15]. "Fetal programming" is a novel concept in reproductive medicine that links various exposures during fetal life to the development of disease later in the life of the offspring [16]. Few studies in this regard have shown some association between maternal hyperthyroidism and the development of attention deficit hyperactivity disorder (ADHD) and epilepsy in offspring of affected mothers [17, 18].

1.6. Diagnosis of Hyperthyroidism in Pregnancy

Hyperthyroidism in pregnancy is diagnosed based on the presence of clinical features as well as laboratory tests. The diagnosis of overt hyperthyroidism during pregnancy is based on the finding of a suppressed (<0.1 mIU/L) or undetectable (<0.01 mIU/L) serum TSH value and a free T4 and/or free T3 (or total T4 and/or total T3) measurement that exceeds the normal range for pregnancy [10]. Once a diagnosis of hyperthyroidism is made, it is essential to differentiate gestational transient hyperthyroidism from GD. Some of the differentiating features of the two conditions are depicted in **Table 1** [11].

When in doubt, TSH receptor antibody (TRAb) testing is done. TRAb may be positive in 96-97% of pregnant women with hyperthyroidism due to GD [19]. Apart from TRAb testing, thyroid ultrasound with a doppler scan may be performed, which may help distinguish GD (high flow) from a sub-acute or painless thyroiditis (low flow). Thyroid scintigraphy, which is usually performed in non-pregnant women to distinguish GD from other causes of thyrotoxicosis, is absolutely contraindicated in pregnancy due to the risk of exposure to ionizing radiation [19].

Table 1. Gestational transient hyperthyroidism versus Graves' disease

Characteristic	Gestational transient hyperthyroidism	Graves' disease
Time of presentation	First trimester	May be diagnosed anytime, usually in the first trimester.
Symptoms and signs	Absent before pregnancy	Might have been present prior to pregnancy
Hyperemesis	More common	No specific relation to hyperemesis
Multiple gestation	More common	No specific relation to multiple gestation
Other manifestations of Graves' disease	Absent	Might be present; for e.g., thyroid eye disease, dermopathy
Family History	Usually unrelated	Maybe present
Severity	Usually mild	Any grade of severity may be present
TSH receptor antibodies	Absent	Present
Course	Self-limited	Unpredictable

2. Management

2.1. Gestational Transient Hyperthyroidism

Anti-thyroid drugs are not usually required as this is a self-limited condition [15]. In case of severe hyperemesis gravidarum, however, supportive treatment to control nausea and vomiting is given, and rarely, hospitalization with administration of intravenous fluids may be required [20]. Thyroid hormones improve gradually as pregnancy progresses. Low dose beta blocker (propranolol) may be given in case of severe symptoms. Thyroid function tests tend to return to normal by 14-18 weeks of gestation [15].

2.2. Graves' Disease in Pregnancy

This consists of addressing the concerns of maternal hyperthyroidism and periodic fetal surveillance.

The aim of treatment is to maintain the total T4/free T4 in the high normal reference range for pregnancy. Anti-thyroid drugs (thionamides) inhibit thyroid hormone synthesis and are the preferred drugs in pregnancy. Propylthiouracil (PTU) is preferred in the 1st trimester as its trans-placental transfer is minimal and is associated with less frequent and milder fetal defects as compared to methimazole (MMI) and carbimazole (CMZ) [21]. Patients on MMI/CMZ are to be switched to PTU if pregnancy is confirmed in the 1st trimester. Subsequently, switching to MMI/CMZ is considered given the risk of hepatotoxicity associated with PTU [22]. Beta blockers (Propranolol 10-40 mg thrice a day) may be used in low doses for symptomatic relief. Methimazole and Carbimazole act by inhibiting thyroxine synthesis. Propylthiouracil, in addition to inhibiting thyroxine synthesis, also inhibits the conversion of T4 to T3. Beta blockers reduce the severity of adrenergic symptoms resulting from the thyrotoxic state. Some of the adverse effects seen with carbimazole and methimazole include agranulocytosis and rash; PTU, in addition may cause fulminant hepatitis. Some of the congenital malformations noted with maternal methimazole in early pregnancy include aplasia cutis, choanal atresia, esophageal atresia, omphalocele, and omphalomesenteric duct anomalies [23]. Some of the rare congenital anomalies observed with PTU include malformation of the face and renal system [24]. Propranolol may cause fetal bradycardia, small for gestational age, and neonatal hypoglycemia.

The initial dose of ATD is decided by the severity of hyperthyroidism and its symptoms. This is as follows:

MMI, 5–30 mg/day (usual dose 10–20 mg/day)
CMZ, 10–40mg/day (usual dose 10-30 mg/day)
PTU, 100–600mg/day (usual dose 200–400 mg/day)

The equivalent potency of MMI to PTU is approximately 1:20 (i.e., 5mg MMI = 100 mg of PTU). Moreover, 10 mg of CMZ is rapidly metabolized to approximately 6 mg of MMI. The half-life of PTU is shorter than that of MMI, and therefore PTU dosing should be split into 2-3 daily doses. MMI is usually given as a single daily dose.

In women treated with ATD, free T4 and TSH are to be monitored every 4 weeks. The primary goal is to maintain free T4 at a high normal reference range. In a woman diagnosed with GD and on ATD, when found to be pregnant, may opt to withhold medications if clinical and biochemical features are suggestive of remission. Following this, her thyroid function tests may be monitored every 2 weeks in the first trimester, and PTU may be initiated if there is evidence of disease recurrence [10]. An approach to hyperthyroidism in pregnancy is shown in Figure 1.

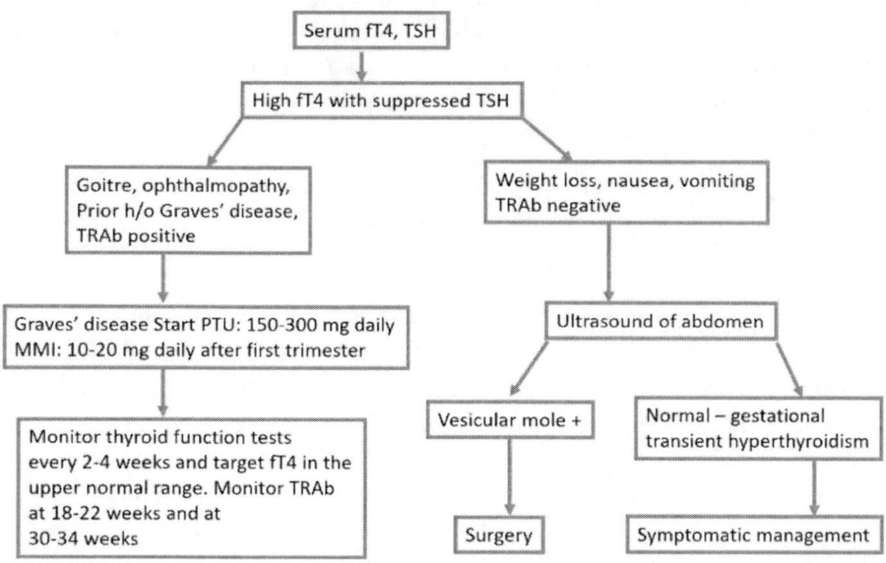

Figure 1. Approach to hyperthyroidism in pregnancy.

As MMI, CMZ, and PTU cross the placental barrier, ATD therapy for maternal hyperthyroidism may potentially modulate fetal thyroid function. As ATDs tend to be more potent in the fetus than in the mother. Therefore, when the mother is made euthyroid, the fetus is often overtreated, leading to hypothyroidism and goiter. In order to avoid deleterious impact on the fetus, the aim of treatment is to maintain the maternal TT4/ FT4 values in the high normal range using the smallest possible dose of ATDs [10].

2.3. Anti-Thyroid Drugs and Congenital Anomalies

Some of the congenital anomalies that have been variously reported with CMZ include aplasia cutis, choanal atresia, patent vitello-intestinal duct, esophageal fistula, omphalocele, imperforate anus, microcolon, gall bladder aplasia, ventricular septal defects, hypoplastic nipples, developmental delay and coloboma of the iris or retina [25]. PTU may be rarely associated with fulminant hepatic failure in the mother. The teratogenic effects associated with PTU use include birth defects of the face and the genito-urinary system, although these are mild compared to the teratogenic effects of CMZ [26]. In a recent meta-analysis that consisted of seven studies, it was found that there was an increased trend of congenital anomalies in hyperthyroid women receiving MMI as compared to healthy women in early pregnancy, while the risk was only slightly increased for PTU as compared to healthy women [27]. Thus, it is reasonable to use PTU as the preferred option in women with hyperthyroidism in early gestation.

2.4. Block-Replace Therapy

The combination of levothyroxine (LT4) and an ATD (block-replace therapy) has not shown to improve the remission rates of GD. The block-replace regimen results in a larger dose of ATD required to maintain the free T4 in the target range. The placenta is more permeable to ATD than LT4, and the fetal thyroid is more sensitive to ATD, this modality of treatment results in fetal hypothyroidism. Therefore, the only indication for such combination therapy during pregnancy lies in the treatment of isolated fetal hyperthyroidism secondary to maternal TRAb production in a mother who has previously received ablative therapy for GD. While the ATD will cross the placenta and lead to the treatment of the fetal hyperthyroidism, the LT4 will serve to maintain maternal euthyroidism [10].

2.5. Radioactive Iodine

Radioactive iodine ablation is absolutely contraindicated in pregnancy due to the risk of radiation exposure to the fetus.

2.6. Surgery

Thyroidectomy in pregnancy may be rarely indicated in cases of uncontrolled hyperthyroidism in spite of being on maximal doses of ATD or in the presence of severe adverse reactions to ATDs. If required, thyroidectomy is considered in the 2nd trimester. In case of poor tolerance to ATD, the preparation for surgery should include a short course of beta-blockers and 50-100 mg/day of potassium iodide solution. Potassium iodide also helps reduce bleeding risk during surgery in case of active thyroid disease. If the maternal TRAb titers are high (> 3 times the upper limit of the reference range), the fetus should be monitored frequently for development of hyperthyroidism even if the mother is rendered euthyroid post thyroidectomy [10].

2.7. TSH Receptor Antibody

The indications for ordering a TRAb test for GD in pregnancy include the following:

- (i) The presence of untreated or ATD-treated hyperthyroidism in pregnancy
- (ii) Prior history of radioiodine ablation or thyroidectomy performed for GD. Any value >5 IU/L or 3 times the upper limit of normal in a mother who previously received radio-iodine ablation for GD mandates close follow-up of the fetus.
- (iii) Previous history of having delivered an infant with neonatal hyperthyroidism
- (iv) To differentiate GD from other causes of thyrotoxicosis

If the TRAb titer done in early pregnancy is found to be low, no further testing is required. If the TRAb in early pregnancy is high, or if the woman requires ATD through mid-gestation, a repeat testing is warranted at 18-22 weeks. If the woman continues to be on ATD through the third trimester or elevated levels of TRAb are detected at 18-22 weeks, a repeat testing is required at weeks 30-34 to assess the need for neonatal monitoring [10].

2.8. Thyroid Storm

Thyroid storm is characterized by a severe, acute exacerbation of the signs and symptoms of hyperthyroidism and is a medical emergency. Patients with hyperthyroidism during pregnancy are 10 times more likely to develop a thyroid storm than during the non-pregnant period. Various stressors such as surgery, childbirth, infection, pre-eclampsia, induced labor and diabetic ketoacidosis may induce maternal thyroid storm.

Precise criteria for thyroid storm were defined by Burch and Wartofsky based on the patient's clinical symptoms, including thermoregulatory and cardiovascular dysfunction, gastrointestinal–hepatic involvement, and central nervous system manifestations [28]. Treatment consists of antithyroid drugs, such as PTU with a saturated solution of potassium iodide and β-blockers which might be aggressively used to reverse the thyrotoxicosis in addition to corticosteroids, oxygen, volume resuscitation, effective temperature control with paracetamol, or cooling blankets, and correction of any underlying dyselectrolytemia [29].

2.9. Autonomous Nodule

Hyperthyroidism due to an autonomous nodule is rare in pregnancy and tends to be less severe as compared to GD. A major difference from GD is the absence of TRAb in this condition. Thus, there is no stimulation of the fetal thyroid and therefore, treatment of the mother to render her euthyroid might cause fetal hypothyroidism. Treatment requires restricting the dose of PTU to the lowest dose possible. Surgery for the autonomous nodule may be considered if there is evidence of fetal hypothyroidism [10].

2.10. Fetal Surveillance

Serial ultrasound examinations are required for the assessment of gestational age, fetal viability, amniotic fluid volume, fetal anatomy, and the detection of fetal malformations. The signs of fetal hyperthyroidism on ultrasound include fetal tachycardia (heart rate >170 bpm, persisting for over 10 minutes), intrauterine growth restriction, |fetal goitre, accelerated bone maturation, signs of congestive heart failure, and fetal hydrops. Serial fetal ultrasound is done once in 4-6 weeks [10].

2.11. Postpartum Period and Lactation

Worsening of hyperthyroidism with a need to increase the dose of ATD or relapse of a previously remitted disease may be expected after delivery. Women need to be warned about this risk, and appropriate monitoring initiated. As far as the management of GD is concerned, both PTU and MMI are detectable in the breast milk of hyperthyroid women on treatment. However, only 0.1-0.2% of an orally administered dose of MMI is excreted in breast milk and a woman on 200 mg thrice daily of PTU secretes 0.149 mg of PTU daily in breast milk. These limits are well below the therapeutic dose [10, 30], and it may be concluded that the use of ATD is safe during lactation.

2.12. Pre-Conceptional Counselling

Ideally, the choice of therapy in the context of pregnancy should be discussed in all women of child-bearing age with GD. It is advisable to postpone pregnancy until a stable euthyroid state is achieved. The use of contraception is recommended till thyroid function tests are under control. A woman who wishes to conceive may be offered definitive treatment in the form of ablative therapy with I-131 (Iodine-131) or thyroidectomy prior to conception [10]. These options may be discussed with the patient in sufficient detail prior to planning a pregnancy in due course.

Conclusion

Hyperthyroidism may be rarely encountered in pregnancy

Management consists of anti-thyroid drugs, beta-blockers and careful attention to foetal well-being

Assessment of TSH receptor antibody testing is undertaken to evaluate the risk of foetal thyrotoxicosis

Uncontrolled hyperthyroidism in pregnancy may lead to adverse maternal and foetal outcomes and therefore warrants close follow-up

References

[1] Nguyen, C. T., Sasso, E. B., Barton, L., and Mestman, J. H. (2018). Graves' hyperthyroidism in pregnancy: a clinical review. *Clin Diabetes Endocrinol.*, 4, 4.

[2] Cignini, P., Cafà, E. V., Giorlandino, C., Capriglione, S., Spata, A., and Dugo, N. (2012). Thyroid physiology and common diseases in pregnancy: review of literature. *J Prenat Med.*, 6(4), 64–71.

[3] Glinoer, D. (1997 Jun). The regulation of thyroid function in pregnancy: pathways of endocrine adaptation from physiology to pathology. *Endocr Rev.*, 18(3), 404–33.

[4] Cole, L. A. (2010 Aug 24). Biological functions of hCG and hCG-related molecules. *Reprod Biol Endocrinol.*, 8, 102.

[5] Soldin, O. P., Chung, S. H., and Colie, C. (2013). The Use of TSH in Determining Thyroid Disease: How Does It Impact the Practice of Medicine in Pregnancy? *J Thyroid Res.*, 2013, 148157.

[6] Fantz, C. R., Dagogo-Jack, S., Ladenson, J. H., and Gronowski, A. M. (1999 Dec). Thyroid function during pregnancy. *Clin Chem.*, 45(12), 2250–8.

[7] McNeil, A. R., and Stanford, P. E. (2015 Nov). Reporting Thyroid Function Tests in Pregnancy. *Clin Biochem Rev.*, 36(4), 109–26.

[8] Sahay, R. K., and Nagesh, V. S. (2012 May). Hypothyroidism in pregnancy. *Indian J Endocrinol Metab.*, 16(3), 364–70.

[9] Moleti, M., Trimarchi, F., and Vermiglio, F. (2014 Jun). Thyroid physiology in pregnancy. *Endocr Pract.*, 20(6), 589–96.

[10] Alexander, E. K., Pearce, E. N., Brent, G. A., Brown, R. S., Chen, H., Dosiou, C., Grobman, W. A., Laurberg, P., Lazarus, J. H., Mandel, S. J., and Peeters, R. P. (2017). Guidelines of the American Thyroid Association for the diagnosis and management of thyroid disease during pregnancy and the postpartum. *Thyroid.*, 2017 Mar 1, 27(3), 315-89.

[11] Cooper, D. S., and Laurberg, P. (2013 Nov). Hyperthyroidism in pregnancy. *Lancet Diabetes Endocrinol.*, 1(3), 238–49.

[12] G Grigoriu, C., Cezar, C., Grigoras, M., Horhoianu, I., Parau, C., Vîrtej, P., Lungu, A., Horhoianu, V., and Poiana, C. (2008 Nov 11). Management of hyperthyroidism in pregnancy. *Journal of Medicine and Life.*, 1(4), 390.

[13] Tingi, E., Syed, A. A., Kyriacou, A., Mastorakos, G., and Kyriacou, A. (2016 Dec). Benign thyroid disease in pregnancy: A state of the art review. *J Clin Transl Endocrinol.*, 6, 37–49.

[14] Prabhu, I. K., and Rosenbaum, A. (2020 Sep 8). Hydatidiform Mole in a Patient With a Concern for Neoplasia: A Case Report. *Cureus.*, 12(9), e10319.

[15] Moleti, M., Di Mauro, M., Sturniolo, G., Russo, M., and Vermiglio, F. (2019 Apr 12). Hyperthyroidism in the pregnant woman: Maternal and fetal aspects. *J Clin Transl Endocrinol.*, 16, 100190.

[16] Andersen, S. L., Olsen, J., and Laurberg, P. (2015 Dec). Foetal programming by maternal thyroid disease. *Clin Endocrinol (Oxf).*, 83(6), 751–8.

[17] Nielsen, T. C., Nassar, N., Shand, A. W., Jones, H., Guastella, A. J., Dale, R. C., and Lain, S. J. (2021 Mar 1). Association of maternal autoimmune disease with attention-deficit/hyperactivity disorder in children. *JAMA pediatrics.*, 175(3), e205487.

[18] Ge, G. M., Leung, M. T., Man, K. K., Leung, W. C., Ip, P., Li, G. H., Wong, I. C., Kung, A. W., and Cheung, C. L. (2020 Dec 1). Maternal thyroid dysfunction during pregnancy and the risk of adverse outcomes in the offspring: a systematic review and meta-analysis. *The Journal of Clinical Endocrinology & Metabolism.*, 105(12), 3821-41.

[19] Bucci, I., Giuliani, C., and Napolitano, G. (2017 Jun 30). Thyroid-Stimulating Hormone Receptor Antibodies in Pregnancy: Clinical Relevance. *Front Endocrinol (Lausanne).*, 8, 137.

[20] Nelson-Piercy, C. (1998 Aug). Treatment of nausea and vomiting in pregnancy. When should it be treated and what can be safely taken? *Drug Saf.*, 19(2), 155–64.

[21] Ramprasad, M., Bhattacharyya, S. S., and Bhattacharyya, A. (2012 Dec). Thyroid disorders in pregnancy. *Indian J Endocrinol Metab.*, 16(Suppl 2), S167-170.

[22] Azizi, F., and Amouzegar, A. (2011 Jun). Management of hyperthyroidism during pregnancy and lactation. *Eur J Endocrinol.*, 164(6), 871–6.

[23] Cassina, M., Donà, M., Di Gianantonio, E., and Clementi, M. (2012 Aug). Pharmacologic treatment of hyperthyroidism during pregnancy. *Birth Defects Res A Clin Mol Teratol.*, 94(8), 612–9.

[24] Yoshihara, A., Noh, J. Y., Watanabe, N., Fukushita, M., Matsumoto, M., Suzuki, N., Hoshiyama, A., Suzuki, A., Mitsumatsu, T., Kinoshita, A., and Mikura K. (2021 Mar). Exposure to propylthiouracil in the first trimester of pregnancy and birth defects: a study at a single institution. *Journal of the Endocrine Society.*, 5(3), bvaa204.

[25] Bowman, P., Osborne, N. J., Sturley, R., and Vaidya, B. (2012 Feb). Carbimazole embryopathy: implications for the choice of antithyroid drugs in pregnancy. *QJM.*, 105(2), 189–93.

[26] Andersen, S. L., Olsen, J., Wu, C. S., and Laurberg, P. (2014 Oct). Severity of birth defects after propylthiouracil exposure in early pregnancy. *Thyroid.*, 24(10), 1533–40.

[27] Li, X., Liu, G. Y., Ma, J. L., and Zhou, L. (2015 Jun). Risk of congenital anomalies associated with antithyroid treatment during pregnancy: a meta-analysis. *Clinics (Sao Paulo).*, 70(6), 453–9.

[28] Burch, H. B., and Wartofsky, L. (1993 Jun). Life-threatening thyrotoxicosis. Thyroid storm. *Endocrinol Metab Clin North Am.*, 22(2), 263–77.

[29] Carroll, R., and Matfin, G. (2010 Jun). Endocrine and metabolic emergencies: thyroid storm. *Ther Adv Endocrinol Metab.*, 1(3), 139–45.

[30] Glatstein, M. M., Garcia-Bournissen, F., Giglio, N., Finkelstein, Y., and Koren, G. (2009 Aug). Pharmacologic treatment of hyperthyroidism during lactation. *Can Fam Physician.*, 55(8), 797–8.

Chapter 13

The Management of Thyrotoxic Storm

Vignesh Gopalakrishnan*

Dr Vignesh's Endocrine and Diabetes Center, Tiruchirappalli, India

Abstract

Thyrotoxic storm (also known as thyrotoxic crisis) is a rare manifestation of thyrotoxicosis which is characterized by multiorgan dysfunction. Presentation is with usual clinical signs and symptoms of thyrotoxicosis along with exaggerated clinical manifestations affecting cardiovascular, gastrointestinal, and central nervous system. Thyrotoxic crisis is either caused by excessive release of thyroid hormones from gland or displacement of free hormones from binding protein along with increased sensitivity to circulating catecholamines and altered peripheral response to thyroid hormone. Thyrotoxic crisis occurs with underlying hyperthyroidism, most commonly Graves' disease. Regardless of the etiology of thyrotoxicosis, its transition to thyrotoxic crisis is precipitated by an underlying factor which can be an infection or any other non-thyroidal illness. Diagnosis is based on clinical features and no specific laboratory test helps to diagnose thyrotoxic storm. Thyroid hormone values usually do not differ from thyrotoxicosis. Based on signs and symptoms, scoring systems have been developed to diagnose this condition in the early phase. Treatment consists of four components – inhibition of thyroid hormone synthesis, blocking the release of stored hormones, prevention of the peripheral conversion of tetraiodothyronine (T4) to triiodothyronine (T3), and supportive care. Clinical improvement usually occurs within 24 hours of initiating therapy. Even with intensive therapy, the mortality rate can be as high as 10-20%. Since thyrotoxic

* Corresponding Author's Email: vigneshmmc2009@gmail.com

In: Understanding and Managing Hyperthyroidism
Editor: Poongkodi Karunakaran
ISBN: 979-8-88697-636-6

crisis carries a high mortality, early clinical recognition is essential to reduce the mortality rate.

Keywords: thyrotoxic storm, thyrotoxic crisis

1. Introduction

Thyrotoxicosis is a clinical syndrome that results when tissues are exposed to supraphysiological levels of thyroid hormones. Thyrotoxic storm (TS) is a sudden exaggerated manifestation of a preexisting thyrotoxic state [1]. Many of the manifestations are related to an increase in oxygen consumption associated with the hypermetabolic state and sympathetic overactivity. The exact pathophysiology of thyroid storm is not fully understood, hypotheses include a rapid rate of increase in circulating thyroid hormone levels, increased responsiveness to catecholamines, or enhanced cellular responses to thyroid hormone. While it is rare in the modern era, mortality remains high, and early therapy improves survival rates.

2. Etiology

Thyrotoxic storm is most commonly associated with preexisting Graves' disease although it can occur in any preexisting hyperthyroid state [2]. TS has been reported in patients who underwent radioiodine treatment [3]. Regardless of the underlying etiology, transition to thyrotoxic storm usually occurs with precipitating factors. Most common precipitating factors include Infection, any acute medical illness, non-thyroid surgery, pregnancy, parturition, emotional stress, iodinated radiographic contrast agents, and sudden cessation of anti-thyroid medicines [4].

3. Pathogenesis

The pathogenesis behind the transition of uncomplicated hyperthyroidism to thyrotoxic storm is unknown. Total thyroid hormone levels are not significantly different from uncomplicated hyperthyroidism, with perhaps one exception, the level of free T4 [5]. But increased hormone levels do clearly play a role in the development of crisis as demonstrated by several scenarios which include post radioiodine therapy, sudden inappropriate withdrawal of thionamide therapy, and iodine induced thyrotoxicosis. Evidence suggested an interaction between the effects of excessive thyroid hormone and catecholamines. Drugs that reduce catecholamine effects like beta-blockers will reduce the severity of clinical manifestations like tachycardia, anxiety, and tremor [6].

4. Clinical Presentation

Typical patients present with usual symptoms of thyrotoxicosis including palpitation, tremor, loss of weight, and increased sweating. Physical examination may reveal goiter, ophthalmopathy (in the presence of Graves' disease), lid lag, hand tremor, and warm and moist skin. With the development of thyrotoxic crisis, clinical features become exaggerated with fever, tachyarrhythmias, jaundice, and CNS involvement. Usually, the transition from hyperthyroidism to thyrotoxic crisis is associated with an underlying precipitating event such as infection, non-thyroid surgery, trauma, burns, or even radiographic iodinated contrast. The most common clinical scenario is sudden inappropriate discontinuation of thionamide drug therapy in a patient with Graves' disease [7]. Thyrotoxic crisis can also occur in patients with toxic multinodular goiter. In elderly patients, the clinical manifestations may be less severe and have been called "apathetic" thyrotoxicosis [8]. If treatment is delayed, it can progress to systemic decompensation and tachyarrhythmias may lead to high output cardiac failure even in patients without underlying cardiac disease. In addition, volume depletion due to fever, diarrhea, or vomiting can lead to hypotension and vascular collapse with shock. Hepatomegaly and jaundice can occur from hepatic congestion. Central nervous system dysfunction includes agitation, panic attack, delirium, psychosis, seizures, and finally coma.

5. Laboratory Findings

As mentioned previously, no definite laboratory cutoff to differentiate thyrotoxicosis from thyrotoxic storm. Serum total and Free T4 and T3 levels are markedly elevated and thyroid stimulating hormone (TSH) will be undetectable. In a critically ill patient with systemic illness, serum T3 levels may be low as seen in lowT3 or euthyroid sick syndrome [9]. Complete blood counts may show relative lymphocytosis in uncomplicated Graves' disease while an underlying infection precipitating TS may present with leukocytosis with shift to left. Hemoconcentration, hypercalcemia and hypokalemia may occur with volume depletion due to recurrent vomiting and diarrhea. Abnormalities in the liver and renal function are directly related to the severity of thyrotoxicosis. Hepatic necrosis or ischemic hepatitis due to heart failure will be associated with elevated serum lactate dehydrogenase (LDH).

6. Diagnosis

Diagnosis of TS is by clinical criteria. Laboratory findings are useful but difficult to distinguish from those in uncomplicated thyrotoxicosis. Based on clinical findings, there are various scoring systems to derive the diagnosis of thyrotoxic crisis [10, 11]. When there is a high index of suspicion, initiation of intensive therapy should be done at the earliest. In order to standardize and objectify thyroid storms, Burch and Wartofsky [10] developed a scoring system assessing degrees of dysfunction in major systems (Table 1). Akamizu et al., [11] developed a scoring system based on elevated serum thyroid hormone levels with CNS and non-CNS manifestations (Table 2). Treatment should not be delayed while determining the etiology of thyrotoxicosis in these patients by measuring thyrotropin receptor antibodies (TRAb) or by doing thyroid scintigraphy.

Table 1. Burch and Wartofsky's diagnostic parameters and scoring points for thyroid storm

Diagnostic parameters	**Scoring points**
1. Thermoregulatory dysfunction Temperature, °C (°F)	
37.2–37.7 (99–99.9)	5
37.7–38.3 (100–100.9)	10
38.3–38.8 (101–101.9)	15
38.9–39.4 (102–102.9)	20
39.4–39.9 (103–103.9)	25
≥40 (≥104.0)	30

Diagnostic parameters	Scoring points
2. Central nervous system effects	
Absent	0
Mild (agitation)	10
Moderate (delirium, psychosis, extreme lethargy)	20
Severe (seizures, coma)	30
3. Gastro-intestinal hepatic dysfunction	
Absent	0
Moderate (diarrhea, nausea/vomiting, abdominal pain)	10
Severe (unexplained jaundice)	20
4. Cardiovascular dysfunction Tachycardia (beats/min):	
90–109	5
110–119	10
120–129	15
130-139	20
≥140	25
5. Congestive heart failure	
Absent	0
Mild (pedal edema)	5
Moderate (bibasilar rales)	10
Severe (pulmonary edema)	15
6. Atrial fibrillation	
Absent	0
Present	10

Scoring system: ≥45, highly suggestive of thyroid storm; 25–44, suggestive of impending storm; <25, unlikely to represent thyroid storm. Table reproduced from: Burch & Wartofsky (1993).

Table 2. Criteria for the diagnosis of thyroid storm by Akamizu et al.,

No.	Diagnostic elements for thyroid storm
1	Elevated serum free T3 or free T4
Signs and symptoms	
2a	CNS Manifestations
	Restlessness Delirium Mental aberration Psychosis Somnolence Lethargy Convulsion Coma Scores 1 or higher on the Japan Coma Scale Scores 14 or lower on the Glasgow Coma Scale

Table 2. (Continued)

No.	Diagnostic elements for thyroid storm	
2b	Non-CNS manifestations	
	Fever	≥38°C
	Tachycardia	≥130 beats/min (includes tachyarrhythmias such as atrial fibrillation)
	CCF	Any one of below: Pulmonary edema Moist rales for more than half the lung field Cardiogenic shock Class IV by the New York Heart Association Class III or higher by the Killip classification
	Gastrointestinal and hepatic	Any one of below: Nausea Vomiting Diarrhea Jaundice Serum bilirubin >3 mg/dL
Diagnosis		
3	Definite	Elevated thyroid hormones (1) + any CNS symptoms in(2a) + one or more of any of non-CNS manifestations in(2b) OR Elevated thyroid hormones (1) + three or more of any of non-CNS manifestations in(2b)
4	Suspect	Elevated thyroid hormones (1) and a combination of two of the following: fever, tachycardia, CCF, or GI/hepatic manifestations OR fulfilling "definite criteria" as above, but raised thyroid hormone could not be determined

Table reproduced by the author with modification and reference based on Akamizu et al., (2012).

7. Treatment

There are four components in the therapy of TS (Table 3). They are: 1) treatment aimed to inhibit thyroid hormone synthesis; 2) block the release of stored hormones; 3) treatment to address the distribution and action of thyroid hormones already in peripheral circulation and 4) symptomatic therapy and treatment of precipitating cause. Treatment should address all four components to avoid fatal outcomes.

7.1. Therapy Directed Against the Thyroid Hormone Synthesis

The thyroid gland in hyperthyroidism is rich in hormone stores and further increased by exposure to excessive amounts of iodine. Blockade of hormone synthesis can be achieved by administration of thionamide antithyroid drugs, such as carbimazole, methimazole, or propylthiouracil (PTU). These drugs can be given via nasogastric tube or via rectum in comatose patients [12, 13]. No intravenous preparations of these agents are available. Higher doses are required in the treatment of TS. PTU has an additional advantage of inhibition of the peripheral conversion of T4 to T3, thereby rapidly lowering the serum T3 concentration [14].

7.2. Inhibit the Release of Stored Hormones

Inorganic iodine given as Lugol's solution or saturated solution of potassium iodide can inhibit the release of stored thyroid hormones into circulation [15]. The sequence of administration of thionamide drugs and iodine is very important. Prior administration of thionamide blocks the hormone synthesis so that the administered iodine will not provide substrate for thyroid hormone production and worsen the TS. In patients allergic to iodine, lithium carbonate may be used to inhibit hormone production and release.

7.3. Reduce the Peripheral Effects of Thyroid Hormone

Beta adrenergic blockers are used to block the effects of thyroid hormones [16-18]. Large doses of propranolol 60 to 120 mg every 6th hour is used in TS. In an intensive care setting, in a comatose patient, short acting beta blockers such as esmolol can be given intravenously [19, 20]. For patients with bronchial asthma or with any other condition where beta blockers are contraindicated, calcium channel blockers such as verapamil can be used. Extraction of thyroid hormones from the blood by peritoneal dialysis, plasmapheresis, or hemoperfusion has been attempted in cases of severe crisis [21, 22].

Table 3. Treatment for thyroid storm

1. Supportive care General: oxygen, cardiac monitoring Fever: external cooling; acetaminophen, 325–650 mg PO/PR every 4–6 Hypovolemia: i.v. isotonic saline (use dextrose containing isotonic saline if blood sugar low)
2. Inhibition of new thyroid hormone synthesis Methimazole, 40 mg given PO as loading dose followed by 20 mg every 4-6 h. Carbimazole 40–60 mg given PO initially, followed by maintenance between 5–20 mg. PTU, a loading dose of 600 mg given PO followed by 200–250 mg every 4-6 h.
3. Inhibition of thyroid hormone release (to be given atleast 1 h after thionamides given) Lugol solution, 8–10 drops PO every 6–8 h or Potassium iodide (SSKI), five drops PO every 6 h or I.v. iopanoic acid, 1 g every 8 h for first 24 h, then 500 mg twice a day or Lithium carbonate (if allergic to iodine or agranulocytosis occurs with thionamides), 300 mg PO every 8 hourly. Serum lithium should be monitored.
4. β-adrenergic receptor blockade Propranolol, i.v. in slow 1–2-mg boluses, may be repeated every 10–15 min until the desired effect is achieved. For less toxic patient, PO dose of 40-80 mg PO q4-6h or Esmolol, 250-500 μg/kg i.v. given in 5 to 10 minutes, then 50–100 μg/kg/min maintenance. or Diltiazem 60-90 mg PO q6-8h (if use of beta-blockers contraindicated)

7.4. Supportive Care

Supportive care includes treatment addressing precipitation events and therapy for systemic decompensation [23]. Precipitating illnesses like ketoacidosis, stroke, or infection may underlie TS. Identification and aggressive management of precipitation illnesses should be done. When no precipitating cause is apparent, a thorough search of infection should be done along with the use of empirical broad-spectrum antibiotics.

Fever should be treated with acetaminophen and external cooling. Aspirin should not be used since it can displace T4 from its binding proteins and increase the free T4 concentration in blood. Volume depletion from fever, vomiting, diarrhea, and sweating should be managed only with fluid replacement. Dextrose normal saline is preferred over saline in order to provide nutritional support. Shock may respond to only fluid replacement and vasopressors are not routinely used due to the sensitivity of these agents and fragile vascular status. Fluids have to be used with caution in elderly patients and patients with poor cardiac reserve. A thyroid storm can accelerate glucocorticoid metabolism and create a relative adrenal insufficiency. Therefore, in cases of thyroid storm associated with severe or refractory hypotension, hydrocortisone (100 mg IV as a loading dose, followed by 100 mg IV every 8 h) may help to correct the hypotension. A stress dose of glucocorticoids should be used in a patient with clinical suspicion of underlying adrenal insufficiency. Glucocorticoids also have an additional benefit of further blockade of peripheral conversion of T4 to T3.

Conclusion

TS is a rare endocrine emergency but is associated with high mortality. It commonly occurs with underlying hyperthyroidism and is precipitated by illness. Prompt identification by clinical features and early intensive treatment improves survival. Treatment should be aimed at blockade of new thyroid hormone synthesis, prevention of release of stored thyroid hormones, reducing the peripheral effects of thyroid hormones and treatment of underlying precipitating illness. During maintenance therapy, measures should be taken to prevent the recurrence of thyroid storm.

References

[1] Nayak, B., Burman, K. D. Thyrotoxicosis and thyroid storm. *Endocrinol Metab Clin North Am* 2006; 35:663–686.

[2] Akamizu, T. Thyroid Storm: A Japanese Perspective. *Thyroid* 2018; 28:32-40.

[3] Rohrs, H. J., 3rd, Silverstein, J. H., Weinstein, D. A., Amdur, R. J., & Haller, M. J. Thyroid storm following radioactive iodine (RAI) therapy for pediatric graves' disease. *Am j Case Rep*. 2014; 15: 212–215.

[4] Ross, D. S., Henry B. Burch, David S. Cooper, M. Carol Greenlee, Peter Laurberg, Ana Luiza Maia, Scott A Rivkees, Mary Samuels, Julie Ann Sosa, Marius N. Stan, Martin A. Walter. 2016 American Thyroid Association Guidelines for Diagnosis and Management of Hyperthyroidism and Other Causes of Thyrotoxicosis. *Thyroid* 2016; 26:1343-1421.

[5] Brooks, M. H., Waldstein, S. S. Free thyroxine concentrations in thyroid storm. *Ann Intern Med.* 1980; 93:694–697.

[6] Feely, J., A. Forrest, A. Gunn, W. Hamilton, I. Stevenson, J. Crooks. Propranolol dosage in thyrotoxicosis. *J Clin Endocrinol Metab* 1980; 51:658–661.

[7] Ylli, D., Klubo-Gwiezdzinska J., Wartofsky L. Thyroid emergencies. *Pol Arch Intern Med.* 2019 Aug 29; 129(7-8):526-534.

[8] Arnold, B. M., Casal G., Higgins H. P. Apathetic thyrotoxicosis. *Can Med Assoc J.* 1974; 111(9):957-958.

[9] Wartofsky, L., Burman K. D. Alterations in thyroid function in patients with systemic illness: the euthyroid sick syndrome. *Endocr Rev* 1982; 3:164–217.

[10] Burch, H. B., Wartofsky, L. Life-threatening thyrotoxicosis: thyroid storm. *Endocrinol Metab Clin North Am* 1993; 22:263–277.

[11] Akamizu, T., Tetsurou Satoh, Osamu Isozaki, Atsushi Suzuki, Shu Wakino, Tadao Iburi, Kumiko Tsuboi, Tsuyoshi Monden, Tsuyoshi Kouki, Hajime Otani, Satoshi Teramukai, Ritei Uehara, Yosikazu Nakamura, Masaki Nagai, Masatomo Mori, Japan Thyroid Association. Diagnostic criteria, clinical features, and incidence of thyroid storm based on nationwide surveys. *Thyroid* 2012; 22:661–679.

[12] Jongjaroenprasert, J. W., W. Akarawut, D. Chantasart, L. Chailurkit, R. Rajatanavin. Rectal administration of propylthiouracil in hyperthyroid patients: comparison of suspension enema and suppository form. *Thyroid* 2002; 12:627–631.

[13] Nareem, N., Miner D. J., Amatruda J. M. Methimazole: an alternative route of administration. *J Clin Endocrinol Metab* 1982; 54:180–181.

[14] Cooper, D. S., V. C. Saxe, M. Meskell, F. Maloof, E. C. Ridgway. Acute effects of propylthiouracil (PTU) on thyroidal iodide organification and peripheral iodothyronine deiodination: correlation with serum PTU levels measured by radioimmunoassay. *J Clin Endocrinol Metab* 1982; 54:101-107.

[15] Wartofsky, L., Ransil B. J., Ingbar S. H. Inhibition by iodine of the release of thyroxine from the thyroid glands of patients with thyrotoxicosis. *J Clin Invest* 1970; 49:78–86.

[16] Das, G., Krieger M. Treatment of thyrotoxic storm with intravenous administration of propranolol. *Ann Intern Med* 1969; 70:985-988.

[17] Feely, J., A. Forrest, A. Gunn, W. Hamilton, I. Stevenson, J. Crooks. Propranolol dosage in thyrotoxicosis. *J Clin Endocrinol Metab* 1980; 51:658–661.

[18] Cooper, D. S., Daniels G. H., Ladenson P. W., Ridgway E. C. Hyperthyroxinemia in patients treated with high-dose propranolol. *Am J Med* 1982; 73:867-871.

[19] Brunette, D. D., Rothong C. Emergency department management of thyrotoxic crisis with esmolol. *Am J Emerg Med* 1991; 9:232-234.

[20] Barbier, G. H., Shettigar U. R., Appunn D. O. Clinical rationale for the use of an ultra-short acting beta-blocker: Esmolol. *Int. J. Clin. Pharmacol.* Ther. 1995; 33: 212–218.

[21] Carhill, A., Gutierrez A., Lakhia R., Nalini R. Surviving the storm: two cases of thyroid storm successfully treated with plasmapheresis. *BMJ Case Rep* 2012 Oct 19; 2012.

[22] Burman, K. D., Yeager H. C., Briggs W. A., Earll J. M., Wartofsky L. Resin hemoperfusion: A method of removing circulating thyroid hormones. *J Clin Endocrinol Metab* 1976; 42:70–78.

[23] Bourcier, S., Maxime Coutrot, Antoine Kimmoun, Romain Sonneville, Etienne de Montmollin, Romain Persichini, David Schnell, Julien Charpentier, Cécile Aubron, Elise Morawiec, Naïke Bigé, Saad Nseir, Nicolas Terzi, Keyvan Razazi, Elie Azoulay, Alexis Ferré, Yacine Tandjaoui-Lambiotte, Olivier Ellrodt, Sami Hraiech, Clément Delmas, François Barbier, Alexandre Lautrette, Nadia Aissaoui, Xavier Repessé, Claire Pichereau, Yoann Zerbib, Jean-Baptiste Lascarrou, Serge Carreira, Danielle Reuter, Aurélien Frérou, Vincent Peigne, Pierre Fillatre, Bruno Megarbane, Guillaume Voiriot, Alain Combes, Matthieu Schmidt. Thyroid Storm in the ICU: A Retrospective Multicenter Study. *Crit Care Med* 2020; 48:83-90.

Chapter 14

Subacute Thyroiditis

Priyadharshini Swaminathan[1,*]
and Premkumar Asokumar[2,†]
[1]SKS Hospital and Postgraduate Institute, Salem, India
[2]Endocrinology, Diaplus Clinics, Salem, India

Abstract

Subacute thyroiditis, also known as Granulomatous thyroiditis, Viral thyroiditis, and de Quervain's thyroiditis, described by Fritz de Quervain in 1905, is an uncommon condition accounting for up to 5% of overall thyroid disorders. It is a self-limiting and remitting inflammatory disease often following an episode of upper respiratory infection. Viral infection provides the antigen either directly or by virus induced host cell damage that binds to HLA molecules on macrophages.

The patient usually presents with anterior neck pain that may radiate to the ipsilateral jaw, throat, ears, and rarely mediastinum. Also, the prodrome of fever, fatigue, myalgia, arthralgia, and anorexia precedes 2 weeks before the illness. Thyroid dysfunction presents with the typical triphasic pattern. The initial phase of thyrotoxicosis wherein damage to thyroid follicles releases the preformed hormone followed by the hypothyroid phase and finally resolving euthyroid phase. The hypothyroid phase is predominantly transient, and permanent hypothyroidism can occur in 25% of patients at the end of 2 years. Diagnosis is based on a complete hemogram showing highly elevated ESR, and CRP. A radionuclide uptake scan is a gold standard in differentiating Graves' disease from subacute thyroiditis, which shows very little uptake. Treatment is predominantly conservative and managed with beta blockers. Antithyroid drugs have no role as there is no increase

* Corresponding Author's Email: dharshini.swaminathan@yahoo.com.

In: Understanding and Managing Hyperthyroidism
Editor: Poongkodi Karunakaran
ISBN: 979-8-88697-636-6

in the production of the hormone. Thyroxine replacement is not needed and the course happens over 3-12 weeks.

Keywords: thyroiditis, subacute thyroiditis

1. Introduction

Subacute thyroiditis, also called by various terminologies including Granulomatous thyroiditis, Giant cell thyroiditis, Noninfectious thyroiditis, viral thyroiditis, pseudotuberculosis, and de Quervain's thyroiditis, is a predominantly self-limiting thyroid disorder. In 1905, Fritz de Quervain differentiated this condition from other thyroiditis by demonstrating granulomatous changes with giant cells as a unique finding after it was described as thyroiditis without abscess formation "thyroiditis akuta simple" in 18 cases by Mygind in 1895. Subacute thyroiditis lasts for weeks to months that may be treated symptomatically. Recurrences have been documented rarely [1].

2. Epidemiology

Subacute thyroiditis is an uncommon condition accounting for up to 5% [2] of overall thyroid disorders and is the most common cause of painful thyroid disease. It has been reported in all age groups, although rare in children and pregnant women. It occurs in temperate zones more frequently during the summer season, despite the lack of its occurrence in tropical and subtropical areas [3]. The seasonal variation coincides with the peak incidence of Echovirus and Coxsackie A&B virus. Women are more commonly affected than men in a ratio of 3: 1 to 6: 1, with a peak incidence in the fourth to the sixth decade. The association of Subacute thyroiditis with SARS-CoV 2 has been reported in a few cases [4, 5].

3. Pathogenesis

Subacute thyroiditis is a self-limiting, remitting inflammatory disease of the thyroid often following an upper respiratory tract infection. Numerous viruses, including influenza, adenovirus, mumps, coxsackievirus, enterovirus, echovirus, Epstein Barr virus, Dengue, Rubella, Hepatitis B, and HIV [6, 7] have been demonstrated to be related. The antecedent history of upper respiratory infection and the detection of viral particles or high viral antibody titers in individuals with Subacute thyroiditis provides evidence for viral and post-viral inflammatory genesis. In addition to various viruses, Chlamydophila psittaci [8] has been linked to Subacute thyroiditis in some cases.

There is a strong association with class 1 major histocompatibility antigen, HLA Bw-35 [9, 10] across many ethnic groups in 72% of cases. HLA-B67 showed a higher incidence of the hypothyroid phase, whereas HLA-B35 progresses from the hyperthyroid phase to the euthyroid phase without hypothyroid interphase. Genetic susceptibility is also evidenced by the occurrence among identical twins [11]. The viral infection provides the antigen, either directly or by virus induced host cell damage, that bind to HLA molecules on macrophages. The resultant antigen -HLA complex that is recognized by the cytotoxic T cells causes damage to the thyroid follicular cells because of molecular mimicry.

There is no association shown between autoimmunity and subacute thyroiditis as anti-TPO, and anti-Tg levels are seen to be normal or transient low titer elevation due to the release of normally sequestered antigens inside the follicles. These autoimmune phenomena could represent a nonspecific response to the inflammatory release of thyroid antigens rather than a specific autoimmune disease. Rare cases of Hashimoto's thyroiditis have been reported, but several cases of the occurrence of Graves' disease after subacute thyroiditis have been published [12]. However, the presence of antithyroid antibodies correlates with a prolonged hypothyroid phase. The pathological findings in histopathology include the infiltration of mononuclear cells and lymphocyte infiltrates in thyroid follicles with patchy disruption of the follicular lining in the early stages. The pathognomonic features include the presence of multinucleated giant cells and granulomatous changes. Interfollicular fibrosis occurs later and eventually returns to normal with no or minimal fibrosis after resolution.

4. Clinical Features

Neck pain is the predominant symptom that may radiate to the ipsilateral jaw, throat, ears, and sometimes mediastinum, which may be sudden or gradual in onset. It may be initially unilateral but later progresses as bilateral pain over the thyroid gland, often termed "migratory thyroiditis" or "creeping thyroiditis." Patients may describe a viral prodrome of fever, fatigue, arthralgia, myalgia and anorexia, and upper respiratory tract infection features in the preceding weeks. Dysphagia may occur and may mislead the diagnosis as pharyngitis. The patient may have low grade fever and rarely present as a Fever of unknown origin. The systemic symptoms gradually progress over 1-2 weeks, and the total duration lasts for 3-6 weeks in general but may last for months. On examination, the thyroid is tender on palpation and moderately enlarged; this may be a diffuse enlargement or asymmetric with palpable nodules.

Recurrence is very rarely documented. Thyroid dysfunction presents with the typical triphasic pattern of hyperthyroidism, a period of hypothyroidism, and a resolving phase to euthyroid status, even though not all patients present with all the phases. Symptomatic hyperthyroidism occurs in up to 60% of [13] patients with a median duration of 43 days and sometimes may precipitate thyrotoxic complications like cardiac arrhythmias, psychosis, and rarely thyroid storm. The hypothyroid phase occurs in 30-60% [14] which in most cases are mild and transient. Permanent hypothyroidism may occur in 15% at the end of 2 years.

5. Diagnostic Evaluation

Routine laboratory evaluation includes Complete blood count, erythrocyte sedimentation rate, C reactive protein, and Thyroid function test. Imaging studies include Radionuclide imaging and thyroid ultrasound. FNAC can be done in specified cases of atypical presentation.

6. Laboratory Tests

Complete blood count may be normal with minimal leukocytosis. Significant leukocytosis is associated with suppurative thyroiditis, which is even rarer. Erythrocyte sedimentation rate is almost always elevated more than 100 mm/hr. C-reactive protein can be elevated during the inflammatory phase in most cases. In the acute phase of illness, there can be hyperthyroxinemia with both T3 and T4 elevation, often high T4 to T3 ratio of about 20:1 [15], indicating the predominance of T4 in the thyroid follicles. Also, in acute illness, deiodinase1 is affected, and hence, poor peripheral conversion of T4 to T3. A discriminatory cut-off value of serum T3 to T4 of 0.4 is used to differentiate between the acute phase of subacute thyroiditis and Graves' disease. There is also a marked increase in thyroglobulin levels as there is damage to thyroid follicles. Anti-thyroid antibodies (anti-thyroid peroxidase & anti-thyroglobulin) are generally absent. Still, transient low titers have been documented [16, 17] and are significantly high and persistent in Hashimoto's thyroiditis which is silent thyroiditis. Positive antithyroid antibodies have been associated with a prolonged hypothyroid phase. Thyroid function tests usually return to normal, but permanent hypothyroidism occurs in up to 15% of patients with severe disease.

There is no specific indication for FNAC thyroid if clinical features and biochemistry correlate. If done, the classical histopathological features include Granuloma formation, in which a central core of degenerative thyroid follicle is surrounded by multinucleate giant cells and epithelioid cells in a background of cellular debris. The "giant cells" consists of masses of colloid surrounded by many histiocytes and are more accurately termed "pseudogiant cells." The lesions are patchy in distribution with infiltration of polymorphonuclear cells into the thyroid follicles in early stages followed by replacement with lymphocytes and macrophages associated with partial or complete loss of colloid. Microabscess formation is seen occasionally. During the recovery phase, the inflammatory changes decrease with a variable amount of interfollicular fibrosis and fibrotic bands.

7. Imaging

Ultrasound thyroid is not a part of the workup for Subacute thyroiditis, but if done may show a hypoechogenic area at the point of thyroid gland tenderness, and it can be enlarged. There are also reported nodules in 70% of patients, which spontaneously resolve [18]. There is also low flow in color doppler sonography in the hyperthyroid phase as there is the destruction of the thyroid follicles that releases the stored T4. Whereas in Graves' disease, there is a diffuse increase in vascularity. The 24-hour Radionuclide uptake scan typically shows markedly reduced or absent uptake termed "low RAIU thyrotoxicosis" during the acute phase, most often $<2\%$, and during the recovery phase, there can be irregular or diffusely increased tracer uptake because of increased iodine trapping [19]. Radionuclide uptake scan is the gold standard investigation in differentiating Subacute thyroiditis from Graves' disease.

8. Differential Diagnosis

The primary differential diagnosis during the acute phase includes suppurative thyroiditis, which is differentiated by the presence of significant leukocytosis. The hyperthyroid phase can be distinguished from Graves' disease by Radionuclide imaging. Sometimes silent thyroiditis or Hashimoto's thyroiditis can be difficult to differentiate, which can be confirmed with specific histopathological findings.

9. Management

The acute thyrotoxic phase is managed symptomatically with beta blockers, and there is no role for antithyroid drugs because there is no increased production of thyroid hormones. Beta blockers can be given for 3-6 weeks; nonselective blockers propranolol and atenolol can also be used. Salicylates and NSAIDs are often used to decrease thyroidal pain in mild to moderate cases. Oral glucocorticoids in moderate to severe cases dramatically relieve pain and swelling within 24-48 hours. The recommended starting dose is 40 mg of Oral Prednisolone and is tapered slowly for 2-4 weeks with symptomatic relief, and doses as low as 15 mg per day are effective in most cases. Tapering can be done by 5 mg every 2 weeks [20]. About 80% of the patients improve within 8 weeks of tapering prednisolone.

A relapse rate of 10-35% [21] has been described in a few studies and rapid dose tapering appeared to be a predictor of relapse. Recently, a therapeutic strategy of intrathyroidal injection of lidocaine and dexamethasone has been described for the treatment of Subacute thyroiditis [22]. Levothyroxine replacement is rarely needed in the early hypothyroid phase as it is usually transient.

Conclusion

Subacute thyroiditis is an uncommon self-limiting, rarely recurrent disease of the thyroid gland where there is the destruction of the thyroid follicles due to a post-viral immune reaction. It is generally managed symptomatically and has complete recovery in almost all cases.

References

[1] Nishihara, E., Hidemi Ohye, Nobuyuki Amino, Kazuna Takata, Takeshi Arishima, Takumi Kudo, Mitsuru Ito, Sumihisa Kubota, Shuji Fukata, and Akira Miyauchi. "Clinical Characteristics of 852 Patients with Subacute Thyroiditis before Treatment." *Internal Medicine (Tokyo, Japan)* 47, no. 8 (2008): 725–29. https://doi.org/10.2169/internalmedicine.47.0740.

[2] "*Subacute Thyroiditis and Acute Infectious Thyroiditis - Werner & Ingbar's The Thyroid: A Fundamental & Clinical Text, 9th Edition.*" Accessed July 26, 2022. https://doctorlib.info/medical/thyroid/39.html.

[3] Martino, E., L. Buratti, L. Bartalena, S. Mariotti, C. Cupini, F. Aghini-Lombardi, and A. Pinchera. "High Prevalence of Subacute Thyroiditis during Summer Season in Italy." *Journal of Endocrinological Investigation* 10, no. 3 (June 1987): 321–23. https://doi.org/10.1007/BF03348138.

[4] Trimboli, P., Chiara Camponovo, Sebastiano Franscella, Enos Bernasconi, and Niccolò Buetti. "Subacute Thyroiditis during the COVID-19 Pandemic: Searching for a Clinical Association with SARS-CoV-2." *International Journal of Endocrinology* 2021 (March 26, 2021): e5588592. https://doi.org/10.1155/2021/5588592.

[5] Bahçecioğlu, A. B., Z. C. Karahan, B. İ. Aydoğan, İ. A. Kalkan, A. Azap, and M. F. Erdoğan. "Subacute Thyroiditis during the COVID-19 Pandemic: A Prospective Study." *Journal of Endocrinological Investigation* 45, no. 4 (2022): 865–74. https://doi.org/10.1007/s40618-021-01718-x.

[6] Sato, M. "Virus-like Particles in the Follicular Epithelium of the Thyroid from a Patient with Subacute Thyroiditis (De Quervain)." *Acta Pathologica Japonica* 25, no. 4 (July 1975): 499–501.

[7] Neupane, B., Sunita Karki, Ekta Tirthani, Nagesh Jadhav, and Nisha Gupta. "A Case of Painless Subacute Thyroiditis Presenting as Fever of Unknown Origin." *Cureus*, May 12, 2022. https://doi.org/10.7759/cureus.24949.

[8] Schofield, P. M., and E. E. Keal. "Subacute Thyroiditis Associated with Chlamydia Psittaci Infection." *Postgraduate Medical Journal* 62, no. 723 (January 1986): 33–34.

[9] Nyulassy, Š., Peter Hnilica, Milan Buc, Milan Guman, Viera Hirschová, and Štefanovic Ján. "Subacute (de Quervain's) Thyroiditis: Association with HLA-Bw35 Antigen and Abnormalities of the Complement System, Immunoglobulins and Other Serum Proteins." *The Journal of Clinical Endocrinology & Metabolism* 45, no. 2 (August 1, 1977): 270–74. https://doi.org/10.1210/jcem-45-2-270.

[10] Stasiak, M., Bogusław Tymoniuk, Bartłomiej Stasiak, and Andrzej Lewiński. "The Risk of Recurrence of Subacute Thyroiditis Is HLA-Dependent." *International*

Journal of Molecular Sciences 20, no. 5 (March 3, 2019): 1089. https://doi.org/10.3390/ijms20051089.

[11] Hamaguchi, E., Yasuyuki Nishimura, Shuichi Kaneko, and Toshinari Takamura. "Subacute Thyroiditis Developed in Identical Twins Two Years Apart." *Endocrine Journal* 52, no. 5 (October 2005): 559–62. https://doi.org/10.1507/endocrj.52.559.

[12] Desailloud, R., and Didier Hober. "Viruses and Thyroiditis: An Update." *Virology Journal* 6, no. 1 (January 12, 2009): 5. https://doi.org/10.1186/1743-422X-6-5.

[13] J. Jacobsen Fatourechi, V., Jaroslaw P. Aniszewski, Guiti Z. Eghbali Fatourechi, Elizabeth J. Atkinson, and Steven. "Clinical Features and Outcome of Subacute Thyroiditis in an Incidence Cohort: Olmsted County, Minnesota, Study." *The Journal of Clinical Endocrinology and Metabolism* 88, no. 5 (May 2003): 2100–2105. https://doi.org/10.1210/jc.2002-021799.

[14] Benbassat, C. A., D. Olchovsky, G. Tsvetov, and I. Shimon. "Subacute Thyroiditis: Clinical Characteristics and Treatment Outcome in Fifty-Six Consecutive Patients Diagnosed between 1999 and 2005." *Journal of Endocrinological Investigation* 30, no. 8 (September 2007): 631–35. https://doi.org/10.1007/BF03347442.

[15] Chen, X., Yulin Zhou, Mengxi Zhou, Qinglei Yin, and Shu Wang. "Diagnostic Values of Free Triiodothyronine and Free Thyroxine and the Ratio of Free Triiodothyronine to Free Thyroxine in Thyrotoxicosis." *International Journal of Endocrinology* 2018 (June 4, 2018): e4836736. https://doi.org/10.1155/2018/4836736.

[16] Stasiak, M., Renata Michalak, Bartłomiej Stasiak, and Andrzej Lewinski. "Clinical Characteristics of Subacute Thyroiditis Is Different than It Used to Be - Current State Based on 15 Years Own Material." *Neuro Endocrinology Letters* 39, no. 7 (February 2019): 489–95.

[17] Alfadda, A. A., Reem M. Sallam, Ghadi E. Elawad, Hisham Aldhukair, and Mossaed M. Alyahya. "Subacute Thyroiditis: Clinical Presentation and Long Term Outcome." *International Journal of Endocrinology* 2014 (2014): 794943. https://doi.org/10.1155/2014/794943.

[18] Cappelli, C., I. Pirola, E. Gandossi, A. M. Formenti, B. Agosti, and M. Castellano. "Ultrasound Findings of Subacute Thyroiditis: A Single Institution Retrospective Review." *Acta Radiologica* (Stockholm, Sweden: 1987) 55, no. 4 (May 2014): 429–33. https://doi.org/10.1177/0284185113498721.

[19] Mariani, G., Massimo Tonacchera, Mariano Grosso, Emilio Fiore, Pierpaolo Falcetta, Lucia Montanelli, Brunella Bagattini, Paolo Vitti, and H. William Strauss. "The Role of Nuclear Medicine in the Clinical Management of Benign Thyroid Disorders, Part 2: Nodular Goiter, Hypothyroidism, and Subacute Thyroiditis." *Journal of Nuclear Medicine: Official Publication, Society of Nuclear Medicine* 62, no. 7 (July 1, 2021): 886–95. https://doi.org/10.2967/jnumed.120.251504.

[20] Kubota, S., Eijun Nishihara, Takumi Kudo, Mitsuru Ito, Nobuyuki Amino, and Akira Miyauchi. "Initial Treatment with 15 Mg of Prednisolone Daily Is Sufficient for Most Patients with Subacute Thyroiditis in Japan." *Thyroid: Official Journal of*

the American Thyroid Association 23, no. 3 (March 2013): 269–72. https://doi.org/10.1089/thy.2012.0459.

[21] Zhang, J., Guoyong Ding, Jingru Li, Xiao Li, Lin Ding, Xiangyun Li, Shuxiang Yang, and Fang Tang. "Risk Factors for Subacute Thyroiditis Recurrence: A Systematic Review and Meta-Analysis of Cohort Studies." *Frontiers in Endocrinology* 12 (2021): 783439. https://doi.org/10.3389/fendo.2021.783439.

[22] Ma, S. G., Feng Bai, and Liang Cheng. "A Novel Treatment for Subacute Thyroiditis: Administration of a Mixture of Lidocaine and Dexamethasone Using an Insulin Pen." *Mayo Clinic Proceedings* 89, no. 6 (June 2014): 861–62. https://doi.org/10.1016/j.mayocp.2014.03.013.

Chapter 15

Hungry Bone Syndrome in Thyrotoxicosis

Poongkodi Karunakaran[1,2,3,*]
Chandrasekaran Maharajan[2,3,†]
and Dorairajan Natarajan[3,‡]
[1]Endocrine Surgery Unit, Government Mohan Kumaramangalam Medical College, Salem, India
[2]Department of Endocrine Surgery, Madras Medical College, Chennai, India
[3]The Tamilnadu Dr. MGR Medical University, Chennai, India

Abstract

Hyperthyroidism is a well-established cause of high bone turnover osteoporosis. Hungry bone syndrome (HBS) is a phenomenon characterized by rapid, profound, and persistent hypocalcemia along with hypomagnesemia and hypophosphatemia due to rapid skeletal remineralization. HBS is a well-known phenomenon after the surgical management of hyperparathyroidism due to the sudden arrest of bone resorption with the rapid decline of parathormone level and restoration of bone mass with calcium influx. Likewise, HBS is well documented after surgical management of hyperthyroidism due to the restoration of loss of bone mass associated with thyrotoxic osteodystrophy. However, a little is known about the occurrence of HBS after treatment of hyperthyroidism with antithyroid drugs and radioactive iodine therapy. This chapter describes the incidence, risk factors, and management of HBS in thyrotoxic patients receiving three different modalities of treatment.

---

* Corresponding Author's Email: poongkodithesurgeon@gmail.com.
† Corresponding Author's Email: profmc@gmail.com.
‡ Corresponding Author's Email: ndr@dr.com.

In: Understanding and Managing Hyperthyroidism
Editor: Poongkodi Karunakaran
ISBN: 979-8-88697-636-6

Keywords: hungry bone syndrome, thyrotoxic osteodystrophy, refractory hypocalcemia

1. Introduction

Thyrotoxicosis is defined as the clinical syndrome of hypermetabolism and hyperactivity that results from excessive circulating levels of free thyroxine (T4) and/or free triiodothyronine (T3). Hyperthyroidism is a subset of thyrotoxicosis characterized by increased synthesis and secretion of thyroid hormones [1]. Thyroid hormones are essential for normal skeletal development and maturation, but untreated thyrotoxicosis can have detrimental effects on bone mineral density (BMD) and increase the fracture risk [2].

1.1. Skeletal Effects of Thyrotoxicosis

The skeleton is a metabolically active tissue in which mineralized bone is continuously remodeled by the coordinated recruitment of osteoclasts and osteoblasts that respectively cause bone resorption and bone formation. Bone resorption lasts for 3-5 weeks, whereas new bone formation is more protracted, lasting for about three months after a reversal phase of two-three weeks. These processes are regulated by autocrine, paracrine, and endocrine pathways. Steroid hormones, particularly glucocorticoids, estrogens, androgens, and vitamin D, are important regulators of bone metabolism. T3 mediates stimulatory action on osteoblasts and has no direct action on osteoclasts [3].

In thyrotoxicosis, the processes of bone resorption, matrix deposition, and mineralization are accelerated, and the activation frequency is increased. Osteoclast and osteoblast activities are both increased (albeit disproportionately), and the duration of the remodeling cycle is reduced by approximately 50%. The uncoupling of osteoclast-osteoblast activation leads to an increase in the ratio of a bone surface undergoing resorption to that undergoing formation. The net result is loss of bone, amounting to approximately 10% of mineralized bone per cycle in severe thyrotoxicosis. In keeping with the increased activity of both osteoclasts and osteoblasts, serum and urinary biochemical markers of bone turnover are high in thyrotoxicosis. They include markers of both bone formation (serum alkaline phosphatase and osteocalcin) and bone resorption (urinary excretion of pyridinoline, deoxypyridinoline cross-links, and hydroxyproline)[4]. Thus, thyrotoxic osteodystrophy is a high bone turnover osteoporosis characterized by decreased BMD (Figure 1). The lack of inhibitory effect of TSH on bone turnover could be another possible reason for high turnover in thyrotoxicosis.

In addition to its direct effects on osteoclast-osteoblast cell function, thyrotoxicosis results in a negative calcium balance. Urinary calcium excretion is increased. Intestinal calcium absorption is decreased, and therefore fecal calcium excretion is increased. The increase in bone resorption raises serum calcium levels, sometimes enough to cause hypercalcemia. Any increase in serum calcium level inhibits parathyroid hormone secretion, thus accounting, at least in part, for the increase in urinary calcium excretion. Another consequence of decreased parathyroid hormone secretion is reduced renal conversion of inactive 25-hydroxyvitamin D (25OHD) to biologically active 1, 25 dihydroxy vitamin D (calcitriol). Reduced activation of vitamin D is exacerbated by enhanced metabolic clearance of vitamin D and its metabolites. Hence, the decrease in vitamin D-mediated intestinal calcium absorption and renal calcium reabsorption. Normal calcium homeostasis and parathyroid hormone secretion are restored after treatment for thyrotoxicosis.

1.2. Skeletal Effects of Childhood Thyrotoxicosis

Thyroid hormones are essential for linear growth and skeletal maturation [2]. T3 regulates chondrocyte differentiation, cartilage matrix synthesis, and mineralization. In children, thyrotoxicosis accelerates skeletal growth. However, advanced bone age causes premature closure of the growth plate, and the ultimate target height is reduced, resulting in short stature. However, studies have demonstrated that timely treatment of thyrotoxicosis with anti-thyroid medication can improve the BMD and revert to the expected growth trajectory.

2. Definition of Hungry Bone Syndrome (HBS)

HBS refers to the phenomenon characterized by rapid, profound, and prolonged hypocalcemia, often associated with hypophosphatemia and hypomagnesemia due to excessive bone remineralization [5]. HBS is caused by the shift of calcium ions along with phosphorous and magnesium into the hungry bones due to the sudden removal of the stimulus for high bone turnover. The high circulating PTH levels fall rapidly after parathyroid adenoma excision in hyperparathyroidism due to its short half-life (3-5 minutes). The rapid fall of PTH leads to sudden arrest of osteoclastic bone resorption in the phase of active bone turnover. This leads to enhanced bone remineralization and manifests as HBS in the immediate postoperative period. The lack of PTH secretion from other suppressed parathyroid glands further exacerbates hypocalcemia. On the other hand, thyrotoxic patients exhibit HBS on the fourth postoperative day, 96 hours after thyroidectomy, with appropriate increases in the PTH levels due to severe hypocalcemia [6]. However, a subset of patients exhibiting HBS after thyroidectomy has hypoparathyroidism due to parathyroid ischemia, devascularization, or unintentional parathyroidectomy during surgery, which further exacerbates hypomagnesemia and refractory hypocalcemia [7, 8].

3. Clinical Manifestation of HBS

Severe hypocalcemia at serum calcium concentration less than 2.1 mmol/L causes neuromuscular irritability. It manifests as acral and perioral paresthesia, positive Chvostek sign and Trousseau sign, carpopedal spasm, laryngospasm, stridor, cardiac arrhythmia, and congestive heart failure [5]. In severe cases, it may lead to seizures, coma, and death.

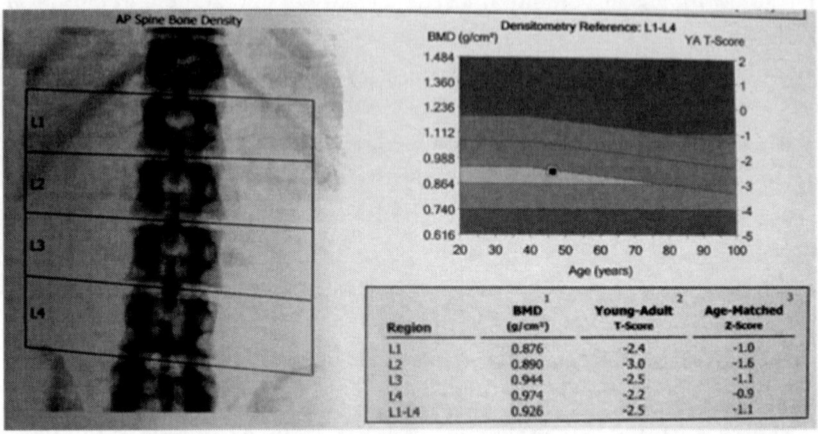

Figure 1. Dual Energy X-ray Absorptiometry scan of Lumbar vertebrae shows reduced bone mineral density and a T-score of -2.5 suggesting severe osteoporosis.

4. Predisposing Risk Factors for HBS

The most critical risk factor for developing HBS is the presence of thyrotoxic osteodystrophy. The greater the severity of osteodystrophy, the higher the risk of developing HBS. This, in turn, depends on the severity and duration of thyrotoxicosis and the magnitude of elevation of thyroid hormones [9]. The degree of severity of osteodystrophy and the speed of recovery of bone loss are the major determinants of the incidence of HBS after treatment of thyrotoxicosis. The rate of recovery of bone loss associated with thyrotoxicosis varies with different treatment modalities such as antithyroid drugs, radioactive iodine (RAI) therapy, or surgery [4, 10]. Studies have shown that recovery of bone mass is prolonged and may be incomplete even after one to four years of treatment with antithyroid drugs or RAI therapy [10]. On the other hand, studies have reported rapid and complete recovery of bone loss associated with thyrotoxicosis as early as six months after thyroidectomy [7, 11]. In a prospective study including 158 subjects, the authors have shown low BMD at diagnosis of hyperthyroidism and improvement with all three modalities of treatment [12]. The study demonstrated an 8.6% improvement of BMD at the spine six months after total thyroidectomy (TT) compared to a 0.9% increase six months post-RAI therapy and an 8.4% increase in BMD hip after TT vs. 2.3% increase post-RAI therapy. The difference was attributed to the quick return of the euthyroid milieu after surgery and hence, bone turnover and restoration of bone mass. In contrast, BMD recovery is delayed after RAI due to the persistent thyrotoxic milieu with the release of the preformed hormone and, later, progressive hypothyroidism [10, 13]. Similarly, the authors have demonstrated that TT for hyperthyroidism elicited the highest BMD recovery in the lumbar vertebrae by 8.3% and was attributed to the increased activation frequency and bone remodeling units in the vertebra, which is cancellous and reflective of bone turnover. In comparison, cortical forearm bone showed the least recovery (3%), while the femur composite of cancellous and cortical bone showed BMD improvement by 7.6% [11]. Additionally, the authors have demonstrated that the incidence of HBS was 32.5% and occurs exclusively in thyrotoxic patients undergoing TT compared to euthyroid controls [7]. The study attributed HBS as the cause of 40% of the cases of post-thyroidectomy hypocalcemia. A few studies have reported HBS in thyrotoxic patients during medical treatment [14]. However, there is a paucity of data on HBS after RAI therapy [10, 15]. Other predisposing factors for developing HBS during treatment include patient-related, surgery-related factors, and certain biochemical parameters. High preoperative calcium, elevated alkaline phosphatase, low magnesium, albumin, and vitamin D deficiency are biochemical predictors of post-thyroidectomy hypocalcemia.

4.1. Preoperative Serum Calcium

Studies have shown that preoperative hypercalcemia is a risk factor for developing HBS after parathyroidectomy in PHPT and post-thyroidectomy in thyrotoxicosis [5]. In contrast to the western population, many of our thyrotoxic patients had low preoperative serum calcium, probably related to the widely prevalent vitamin D deficiency in our Indian population [7, 11].

4.2. High Serum Alkaline Phosphatase

Serum alkaline phosphatase is a marker of bone turnover and bone formation. Studies have shown that vertebral osteoporosis with the concomitant two-fold elevation of alkaline phosphatase in thyrotoxic patients at diagnosis is associated with a higher incidence of HBS during treatment [7, 16]. Studies have shown persistent elevation of alkaline phosphatase even after one to four years of treatment with antithyroid drugs and a few episodes of HBS [17].

4.3. Preoperative Low Magnesium and Albumin

HBS is associated with the influx of calcium and phosphorous along with magnesium during bone remineralization after treatment of hyperthyroidism. Hence, pre-existing low serum magnesium concentration, particularly in young women, exacerbates the phenomenon. Studies have shown that both the low serum magnesium and its rapid fall within 48-hour after surgery in Graves' disease is an important predisposing factor for HBS [7, 18]. Moreover, bivalent magnesium cation is an allosteric modulator of calcium-sensing receptors, and hypomagnesemia per se causes refractory hypocalcemia. Additionally, hypomagnesemia decreases the PTH release and its target organ responsiveness, further exacerbating refractory hypocalcemia [8, 19]. Hypoalbuminemia is associated with increased risk of postoperative hypocalcemia after thyroidectomy.

4.4. Vitamin D Deficiency

Vitamin D is an independent predictor of bone health, and vitamin D deficiency is associated with reduced BMD in thyrotoxicosis [20]. However, the impact of vitamin D deficiency on BMD recovery and risk for HBS is controversially reported [18, 21]. A recent case report has shown that severe vitamin D deficiency is a risk factor for developing HBS after antithyroid therapy for thyrotoxicosis. On the contrary, in a prior report, the author has shown that 25OHD was a poor predictor of post-thyroidectomy hypocalcemia in thyrotoxic subjects [22].

4.5. Patient-Related Risk Factors

Some studies report that advancing age and post-menopausal women are predisposing patient-related risk factors for developing HBS, while others refute [18, 23, 24].

4.5.1. Rapid Restoration of Euthyroid Status

Rapid preparation of thyrotoxic patients with high-dose antithyroid drugs or steroids with or without beta-blockers to achieve euthyroid status is likely to increase the risk of HBS after treatment, both medical and surgical management. In thyrotoxic high bone-turnover osteopenia, osteoblastic bone formation lags behind bone resorption by 12 weeks or more [3]. It is possible that with the restoration of euthyroid status and normal bone turnover, there is rapid skeletal remineralization of expanded remodeling space, increasing the risk of HBS.

4.6. Surgery-Related Risk Factors

Rapid preparation for surgery, prolonged operative duration and consequent intraoperative fluid dynamics, meticulous handling, and the number of remaining functional parathyroid glands are surgery-related factors likely to increase the risk of HBS [18, 25].

5. Biochemical Changes in HBS

- Serum corrected serum calcium falls below 8 mg/dl within 48-72 hours, but further fall occurs after the fourth postoperative day in patients with HBS
- Decline of serum phosphate levels postoperatively
- Hypomagnesaemia
- Two-fold elevation of serum alkaline phosphatase
- Rise in PTH levels. In contrast to PHPT, hypocalcemia of HBS in thyrotoxicosis is characterized by appropriate increases in parathormone levels. However, in a subset of patients exhibiting HBS after thyroidectomy, PTH levels may fall due to postoperative hypoparathyroidism resulting from devascularization or accidental parathyroidectomy.

6. Management of HBS

The management of HBS consists of short-term goals to replenish the circulating calcium deficit and long-term goals to normalize bone turnover and achieve complete bone remineralization. Acute hypocalcemia is treated intravenously with 10 ml of 10% calcium gluconate (90 mg of elemental calcium per 10 mL ampoule) over 10 minutes. Persistent hypocalcemia is treated with 10% calcium gluconate infusion at a rate of 0.5-2.0 mg/kg/hour until serum corrected calcium maintains in the low normal range. Adverse effects include cardiac arrhythmia, local irritation, vasculitis with extravasation of calcium chloride, and ectopic calcification with calcium phosphate crystal deposition. Oral calcium supplementation up to 3g per day with calcitriol (0.25 to 1 mcg/day) is required. Refractory hypocalcemia, resistant to intravenous calcium therapy, requires judicious correction of magnesium deficiency with intravenous magnesium sulfate or oral doses of magnesium oxide. Simultaneous rapid calcium and magnesium infusion can form calcium complexes and precipitate tetany. Studies have shown that prolonged duration of surgery and the consequent intraoperative hemodynamic changes like hemodilution and hypoalbuminemia can increase the incidence of hypomagnesemic hypocalcemia syndrome after TT [8]. Supportive management will facilitate the amelioration of these symptoms. Long-term oral calcium therapy with or without vitamin D analogs may be required to maintain eucalcemia and complete bone recovery. The utility of anti-resorption agents, including bisphosphonates and denosumab, in the management of thyrotoxic osteodystrophy and HBS, needs elucidation. Newer recombinant human PTH analogs, namely rhPTH (1-34) and rhPTH (1-84), have shown promising results in osteoporosis and postoperative hypoparathyroidism [26]. The utility of PTH analogs in thyrotoxic HBS management is the future research direction.

Conclusion

The hungry bone syndrome is a life-threatening hypocalcemic phenomenon due to rapid skeletal remineralization, not uncommon after treatment of hyperthyroidism. HBS occurs exclusively in thyrotoxic patients undergoing total thyroidectomy, with a registered incidence of 32.5%. Nevertheless, a few cases have been reported with other forms of therapy. Vertebral osteoporosis with concomitant serum alkaline phosphatase elevation, rapid restoration of euthyroid status, and steep slope of serum magnesium within 48 hours after surgery are likely to increase the risk of HBS. The treatment goals are to replenish the circulating mineral deficits and normalize bone turnover.

References

[1] de Leo S., Lee S. Y., Braverman L. E. Hyperthyroidism. The *Lancet* 2016;388:906–18. https://doi.org/10.1016/S0140-6736(16)00278-6.

[2] Bassett J. H. D., Williams G. R. Role of Thyroid Hormones in Skeletal Development and Bone Maintenance. *Endocrine Reviews* 2016;37:135–87. https://doi.org/10.1210/er.2015-1106.

[3] Freudenthal B., Watts L., Williams G. R., Bassett J. H. D. The skeletal system in thyrotoxcosis. In: Braverman L. E., Cooper D. S., Kopp P., editors. *Werner & Ingbar's The Thyroid: A Fundamental and Clinical Text,* vol. 1. 11th ed., Philadelphia: Lippincott Williams & Wilkins (LWW); 2020, p. 454–62.

[4] Pantazi H., Papapetrou P. D. Changes in parameters of bone and mineral metabolism during therapy for hyperthyroidism. *Journal of Clinical Endocrinology and Metabolism* 2000;85:1099–106. https://doi.org/10.1210/jc.85.3.1099.

[5] Witteveen J. E., van Thiel S., Romijn J. A., Hamdy N. A. Hungry bone syndrome: still a challenge in the post-operative management of primary hyperparathyroidism: a systematic review of the literature. *European Journal of Endocrinology/European Federation of Endocrine Societies* 2013;168. https://doi.org/10.1530/EJE-12-0528.

[6] Dembinski T. C., Yatscoff R. W., Blandford D. E. Thyrotoxicosis and Hungry Bone Syndrome-A cause of posttreatment hypocalcemia. *Clinical Biochemistry* 1994;27:69–74. https://doi.org/10.1016/0009-9120(94)90014-0.

[7] Karunakaran P., Maharajan C., Ramalingam S., Rachmadugu S. V. Is hungry bone syndrome a cause of postoperative hypocalcemia after total thyroidectomy in thyrotoxicosis? A prospective study with bone mineral density correlation. *Surgery* (United States) 2018;163:367–72. https://doi.org/10.1016/j.surg.2017.09.008.

[8] Wilson R. B., Erskine C., Crowe P. J. Hypomagnesemia and hypocalcemia after thyroidectomy: Prospective study. *World Journal of Surgery* 2000;24:722–6. https://doi.org/10.1007/s002689910116.

[9] el Hadidy E. H. M., Ghonaim M., el Gawad S. S. A., el Atta M. A. Impact of severity, duration, and etiology of hyperthyroidism on bone turnover markers and bone mineral density in men. *BMC Endocrine Disorders* 2011;11. https://doi.org/10.1186/1472-6823-11-15.

[10] Langdahl B. L., Loft A. G., Eriksen E. F., Mosekilde L., Charles P., Gitte A. Bone mass, bone turnover, calcium homeostasis, and body composition in surgically and radioiodine-treated former hyperthyroid patients. *Thyroid* 1996;6:169–75. https://doi.org/10.1089/thy.1996.6.169.

[11] Karunakaran P., Maharajan C., Mohamed K. N., Rachamadugu S. V. Rapid restoration of bone mass after surgical management of hyperthyroidism: A prospective case control study in Southern India. *Surgery* 2016;159:771–6. https://doi.org/10.1016/j.surg.2015.10.002.

[12] Karunakaran P., Maharajan C., Chockalingam R., Asokumar P., Koramadai Karuppusamy K., Sadasivam V. The effect of total thyroidectomy on the recovery of bone mineral density in subjects with hyperthyroidism. *Surgery* (United States) 2019;165:80–4. https://doi.org/10.1016/j.surg.2018.05.082.

[13] Rosario P. W. Radioiodine therapy in elderly patients with subclinical hyperthyroidism due to non-voluminous nodular goiter and its effect on bone metabolism. *Arquivos Brasileiros de Endocrinologia & Metabologia* 2013;57:144–7. https://doi.org/10.1590/S0004-27302013000200008.

[14] Grieff M. The Hungry Bone Syndrome after Medical Treatment of Thyrotoxicosis. *Annals of Internal Medicine* 2003;139:706. https://doi.org/10.7326/0003-4819-139-8-200310210-00027.

[15] Lazareva O., Panayiotopoulos A., Kazachkova I., Jacobson-Dickman E. A teenage boy with hypocalcemia after radioablation for Graves' disease. *Journal of Pediatric Endocrinology and Metabolism* 2014;27. https://doi.org/10.1515/jpem-2013-0322.

[16] Yamashita H., Noguchi S., Murakami T., Uchino S., Watanabe S., Ohshima A., Toda M., Yamashita H., Kawamoto H. Predictive risk factors for postoperative tetany in female patients with Graves' disease. *Journal of the American College of Surgeons*. 2001 Apr 1;192(4):465-8.

[17] Udayakumar N., Chandrasekaran M., Rasheed M. H., Suresh R. V. Evaluation of bone mineral density in thyrotoxicosis. *Singapore Medical Journal* 2006;47:947–50.

[18] Edafe O., Antakia R., Laskar N., Uttley L., Balasubramanian S. P. Systematic review and meta-analysis of predictors of post-thyroidectomy hypocalcaemia. *British Journal of Surgery* 2014;101:307–20. https://doi.org/10.1002/bjs.9384.

[19] Karunakaran P., Abraham D., Devadas G., Hussain Z., Kanakasabapathi R. The Effect of Hypomagnesemia on Refractory Hypocalcemia after Total Thyroidectomy: A Single-Center Prospective Cohort Study. *Indian Journal of Endocrinology and Metabolism* 2020;24. https://doi.org/10.4103/ijem.IJEM_681_20.

[20] Karunakaran P., Abraham D. T., Devadas G., Hussain Z., Kanakasabapathi R. Is Preoperative Vitamin D Deficiency a Predictor of Transient and Permanent Hypocalcemia After Total Thyroidectomy? A Cohort Study in a Tertiary Care Hospital. *Indian Journal of Surgery* 2021. https://doi.org/10.1007/s12262-021-03183-5.

[21] Manzini G., Malhofer F., Weber T. Can preoperative vitamin D deficiency predict postoperative hypoparathyroidism following thyroid surgery? *Langenbeck's Archives of Surgery* 2019;404:55–61. https://doi.org/10.1007/s00423-019-01748-3.

[22] Karunakaran P., Abraham D. T. The utility of serum 25-hydroxyvitamin D in predicting post-thyroidectomy hypocalcemia in thyrotoxic subjects: a single-center cohort study. *International Surgery Journal* 2020;7. https://doi.org/10.18203/2349-2902.isj20205359.

[23] Serraclara A., Jódar E., Sarabia F., Hawkins F. Bone mass after long-term euthyroidism in former hyperthyroid women treated with131I: Influence of menopausal status. *Journal of Clinical Densitometry* 2001;4:249–55. https://doi.org/10.1385/JCD:4:3:249.

[24] Puzziello A., Rosato L., Innaro N., Orlando G., Avenia N., Perigli G., Calò P. G., De Palma M. Hypocalcemia following thyroid surgery: incidence and risk factors. A longitudinal multicenter study comprising 2,631 patients. *Endocrine*. 2014 Nov;47(2):537-42.

[25] Karunakaran P., Abraham D. T., Devadas G., Ramalingam S., Balu S., Hussain Z. The impact of operative duration and intraoperative fluid dynamics on postoperative hypocalcemia after total thyroidectomy: a prospective non-randomized study. *Langenbeck's Archives of Surgery* 2021;406:1211–21. https://doi.org/10.1007/s00423-020-02013-8.

[26] Sikjaer T., Rejnmark L., Mosekilde L. PTH Treatment in Hypoparathyroidism. *Current Drug Safety* 2011;6:89–99. https://doi.org/10.2174/157488611795684631.

Chapter 16

Drug-Induced Hyperthyroidism

K. V. S. Hari Kumar[*], MD, DNB
Endocrinology, MAGNA Clinic, Hyderabad, India

Abstract

The thyroid gland is one of the endocrine glands with a rich blood supply resulting in exposure to the circulating pharmaceutical agents in higher concentrations. Iodine is the primary ingredient of thyroid hormones, and iodine-induced hyperthyroidism is observed in areas with iodine deficiency and endemic goiter. Amiodarone is a common antiarrhythmic agent, with iodine being the principal constituent, affecting the thyroid gland's functioning. Thyroid hormone overdose is the commonest cause of drug-induced thyrotoxicosis observed in clinical practice. Many drugs lead to inflammatory destruction of the thyroid parenchyma leading to transient thyrotoxicosis with associated symptoms. In this chapter, I shall present a brief overview of the drugs leading to thyrotoxicosis and the relevant clinical evaluation, including the management.

Keywords: drug-induced hyperthyroidism, drug-induced thyrotoxicosis, iodine-induced hyperthyroidism

1. Introduction

The thyroid gland has a rich blood supply and is exposed to a reasonable concentration of pharmacological agents in blood circulation. Iodine is the

[*] Corresponding Author's Email: hariendo@gmail.com.

In: Understanding and Managing Hyperthyroidism
Editor: Poongkodi Karunakaran
ISBN: 979-8-88697-636-6

principal constituent of thyroid hormone synthesis, and consumption of iodine-containing preparations alters thyroid hormone synthesis. Other drugs may result in the inflammatory destruction of the thyroid, leading to transient thyrotoxicosis followed by remission or hypothyroidism [1]. In clinical practice, an overdose of thyroxine is the commonest cause of drug-induced thyrotoxicosis. This section will discuss the issues concerning drug-induced hyperthyroidism and appropriate management options.

2. Iodine

Iodine-induced hyperthyroidism (also known as Jod – Basedow phenomenon) is rarely seen in the current world and is often self-limiting. Elderly patients with autonomously functioning nodules and early Graves' disease (GD) are predisposed to developing iodine-induced hyperthyroidism. Patients in remission after managing GD are also susceptible to this condition. The prevalence of autonomous thyroid nodules increases in patients living in iodine deficiency areas, and sudden intake of excess iodine in these patients may trigger hyperthyroidism [2]. A recent meta-analysis has suggested that iodine-induced hyperthyroidism is mild and often subclinical. The risk of developing overt thyrotoxicosis after iodine contrast exposure is too low to justify any prophylactic use of antithyroid drugs.

Treating iodine-induced hyperthyroidism primarily avoids further exposure to iodine and symptomatic relief with beta-blockers. Antithyroid drugs are required in rare situations of severe thyrotoxicosis, and higher doses may be needed in these conditions. Radioiodine therapy may only be beneficial once the excess iodine load is cleared. The clearance of the iodine load may be estimated by monitoring the urinary iodine levels.

3. Amiodarone

Amiodarone is an antiarrhythmic drug with 37% of iodine as the primary constituent. This results in the consumption of extra iodine by the patients and may have different consequences depending on the patient's underlying status. Amiodarone-induced thyrotoxicosis (AIT) is seen in about 6 to 10% of patients, depending on the underlying iodine status of the population [3]. There are two distinct types of AIT, type 1 being similar to iodine-induced hyperthyroidism, whereas type 2 is due to thyrocyte damage induced by the drug.

It is recommended to do a thyroid function before the starting of amiodarone in patients and serial monitoring of the thyroid functions while the patient is using the drug. The decision to stop amiodarone should be taken in consultation with the cardiologist. It is advisable not to stop the medication as this may worsen the underlying cardiac condition. Antithyroid drugs treat type 1 AIT, and Type 2 AIT is treated using a short course of glucocorticoids. Combination therapy is used in certain patients when the distinction is unclear and to benefit from the peripheral antithyroid effects of glucocorticoid drugs. In patients who do not respond to the combination therapy, therapeutic options are limited between either thyroidectomy or stopping the amiodarone.

4. Thyroxine

Excessive consumption of thyroxine, intentionally or accidentally, is the common cause of drug-induced thyrotoxicosis. Frequently thyroid hormones have been used to increase the metabolism and are abused as a weight loss agent by unqualified practitioners. Hamburger thyrotoxicosis is the term that denotes the accidental consumption of an excessive quantity of meat contaminated with the animal thyroid leading to thyrotoxicosis.

The evaluation of clandestine thyroxine ingestion is often tricky and is aided by the absence of goiter, reduced thyroid uptake, and suppressed thyroglobulin levels. Thyroid sonography and thyroid antibodies have a minimal role in evaluating this condition. Fecal thyroxine levels help identify concealed ingestion, and these patients are given psychotherapy along with a stoppage of thyroxine consumption [4]. Occasionally patients may require cholestyramine or charcoal hemoperfusion to clear the circulating level of excess thyroid hormones [5].

5. Lithium

Lithium is a drug used to treat mania and bipolar affective disorder. Lithium is concentrated by the thyroid and inhibits the release of thyroid hormones leading to goitrous hypothyroidism. Occasionally, the drug may result in thyrotoxicosis by various mechanisms, including the formation of thyroid-stimulating autoantibodies, thyroiditis, and escape of the phenomenon of the thyroid hormones leading to the release of excess hormones. The relation between lithium and thyrotoxicosis is bi-directional in which thyrotoxicosis itself may augment the lithium toxicity by increasing the reabsorption of the lithium in the proximal tubule, thereby reducing the fractional excretion of the lithium [6]. In certain situations, it is difficult to distinguish between the psychological features due to the underlying disease, lithium toxicity, or impending thyroid storm. The management is to stop the lithium and select any other psychoactive drug that does not affect thyroid function.

6. Others

Many other drugs increase the risk of destructive thyrotoxicosis in patients. The list includes interferon-α, interleukin-2, and tyrosine kinase inhibitors like Sunitinib, Sorafenib, and Nilotinib [7]. The patients prescribed these drugs are advised baseline thyroid function screening and regular monitoring at 3-6 monthly intervals to identify thyroid dysfunction at an early stage. Most of these patients are treated symptomatically with beta-blockers, and in a few resistant cases, glucocorticoids may be required.

Conclusion

To conclude, drug-induced hyperthyroidism is an entity that requires a detailed history to identify the offending drug. The past may not be forthcoming and diagnostic aids are needed in some instances of factitious thyrotoxicosis. In most cases, withdrawal of the offending drug is sufficient for the management. However, in patients with severe symptoms, beta-blockers, antithyroid drugs, and even glucocorticoids are recommended.

References

[1] Barbesino G. Drugs affecting thyroid function. *Thyroid,* 2010; 20:763-770.
[2] Roti E, Uberti ED. Iodine excess and hyperthyroidism. *Thyroid,* 2001; 11(5):493-500.
[3] Basaria S, Cooper DS. Amiodarone and the thyroid. *Am J Med,* 2005; 118:706-714.

[4] Bouillon R, Verresen L, Staels F, Bex M, De Vos P, De Roo M. The measurement of fecal thyroxine in the diagnosis of thyrotoxicosis is factitive. *Thyroid,* 1993; 3:101-3.

[5] Kreisner E, Lutzky M, Gross JL. Charcoal hemoperfusion in the treatment of levothyroxine intoxication. *Thyroid,* 2010; 20: 209-212.

[6] Oakley PW, Dawson AH, Whyte IM. Lithium: Thyroid effects and altered renal handling. *J Toxicol Clin Toxicol*, 2000; 38: 333-7.

[7] Carella C, Mazziotti G, Amato G, Braverman LE, Roti E. Clinical review 169: Interferon-alpha-related thyroid disease: Pathophysiological, epidemiological and clinical aspects. *J Clin Endocrinol Metab,* 2004; 89: 3656-3661.

Index

I

M

N

O

P

R

S

T

About the Editor

Poongkodi Karunakaran, MS, MCh, PhD, Senior Civil Surgeon & Assistant Professor of Endocrine Surgery, Principal Investigator, ICMR Extramural Scheme, Government Mohan Kumaramangalam Medical College, Salem, Madras Medical College, Chennai, India.

Email: poongkodithesurgeon@gmail.com